Porcelain Laminate Veneers

David A. Garber, D.M.D. ● Ronald E. Goldstein, D.D.S. ● Ronald A. Feinman, D.M.D.

Porcelain Laminate Veneers

David A. Garber, D.M.D., B.D.S.

Clinical Professor of Periodontics
Medical College of Georgia

Special Lecturer in Esthetic Dentistry
Emory University School of Dentistry

Private Practice, Atlanta, Georgia

Ronald E. Goldstein, D.D.S.

Clinical Professor of Restorative Dentistry
Medical College of Georgia

Special Lecturer in Esthetic Dentistry
Emory University School of Dentistry

Associate Clinical Professor of Continuing Education
Boston University Goldman School of Graduate Dentistry

Private Practice, Atlanta, Georgia

Ronald A. Feinman, D.M.D.

Special Lecturer in Esthetic Dentistry
Emory University School of Dentistry

Private Practice, Atlanta, Georgia

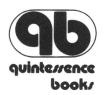
**quintessence
books**

Quintessence Publishing Co., Inc. 1988
Chicago, London, Berlin, Tokyo, São Paulo, Hong Kong

Library of Congress Cataloging-in-Publication Data

Garber, David A.
  Porcelain laminate veneers.

    Includes bibliographies and index.
    1. Dental ceramics. 2. Dental veneers.
3. Dentistry—Aesthetics. I. Goldstein, Ronald E.
II. Feinman, Ronald A. III. Title. [DNLM: 1. Dental
Porcelain. 2. Dental Veneers. 3. Esthetics, Dental.
WU 190 G213p]
RK655.G34 1988   617.6'95   87-29272
ISBN 0-86715-194-3

Lithography: Industrie- und Presseklischee, Berlin
Composition: Graphic World, Inc., St. Louis, MO
Printing and binding: The Ovid Bell Press, Inc., Fulton, MO
Printed in U.S.A.

Contents

Contributors

Pinhas Adar, C.D.T.

Atlanta, Georgia

Thomas Greggs, C.D.T.

Wheaton, Illinois

Harald O. Heymann, D.D.S., M.Ed.

Associate Professor
Department of Operative Dentistry
University of North Carolina School of Dentistry

Dan Nathanson, D.M.D., M.S.D.

Director of Continuing Education Division
Professor and Chairman
Department of Biomaterials
Boston University Goldman School of Graduate Dentistry

Dedication

A captivating smile showing an even row of natural, gleaming white teeth is a major factor in achieving that elusive dominant characteristic known as personality. This entails a lack of an inferiority complex due to crooked, unsightly teeth, which during speech causes a hand to be raised to cover the mouth or manipulation of the lips in an unnatural manner to make up for the defect. It is this lack of confidence in the dental equipment which often spells the difference in success and failure on the part of many people. . . .

This quote is from a paper by Charles Pincus, D.D.S., read before the California State Dental Association in April, 1937, some nine years after he began to develop concepts of dental esthetics while working with the movie industry. His creativity included the first recorded use of porcelain laminates to temporarily cover esthetic deformities of actors while they were being filmed.

We were proud to be his students and his friends and consider it fitting to dedicate this text to his memory.

Preface

The advent of etching enamel started what has become the most overwhelming surge of interest in dentistry since the invention of high-speed cutting instruments. Many generations of bonded composite resins have chipped, fractured, or discolored—despite the retentive surface of enamel. Thus, a need developed for a better solution, and porcelain laminates evolved. No other technique in dentistry has enjoyed such rapid, wide-spread utilization and at the same time proven itself with such predictable esthetic results.

The emerging importance of porcelain laminate veneers in restorative dentistry has created a void in the dental literature. Not only are the "how, when, and why's" essential to an understanding, but also the role of this new restorative combined with other treatments.

We have attempted to produce a thorough look at one of the newest and most exciting clinical approaches to restorative dentistry. In doing so, it is our hope that it will fill a missing link in the dental literature.

Foreword

Rarely does it become possible for an individual who has been involved in the early research and development phase of a new technique to have the opportunity to see it become one of the most widely used and accepted dental restorative procedures in the world. The concepts of bonded esthetic dentistry and laminate veneers is truly exciting and holds unforetold promise for the future. It is also rare to see a new technique discussed with such clarity in an easily understood and practical fashion for the dental practitioner.

Dr. David A. Garber and his partners, Drs. Ronald E. Goldstein and Ronald A. Feinman, are among the world's finest clinicians. They have indeed developed another excellent book for the dental profession. This book should occupy a favored place in the library of every dental practitioner and educator throughout the globe.

I am pleased to have been asked to write the foreword for this book and must suggest to the reader that they are in for a real surprise if they anticipated a dull or dry treatise as so many "how to" dental books have been written. The text grabs the interest and imagination of the reader right from the beginning of the first chapter through to the last. The authors instill their own particular flavor of excitement and energy for esthetic dentistry, and their enthusiasm is reflected in every word and illustration.

The first chapter deals with the history of bonding procedures in dentistry and the development of laminate veneers. This chapter explains the chain of events that led to the present state of the art in esthetic dentistry. It will leave the reader anticipating the exciting future that the field will enjoy.

Many dentists may feel an "either/or" relationship to any particular dental procedure, but these clinicians clearly explain the "whys" in the chapter on indications and contraindications for laminate veneers. They have illustrated their comments with a variety of cases that they have seen.

In the approach to the technical side, they do not burden the reader but instead delight them with the reasons for success or failure with the laminate veneer restoration. The no-nonsense approach to the basics of material science leaves the clinician well founded for success with the technique.

The explanations of the dental biomaterials involved in this technique and of the preparations for the laminate veneers are well done, as is the relevant discussion of clinical procedures in the dental office, which lays a solid foundation for the laboratory technician.

If the dentist finds the chapters on laboratory fabrication of laminate veneers and on the special effects that this procedure offers to be exciting, then I suspect that these chapters will be of special interest to the truly artistic dental laboratory technician. The authors develop a theme of artistic dentistry and its expressions through laminate veneers in a manner that should challenge every dentist and dental technician.

In many books placement procedures and techniques for restorations are explained vaguely, which frequently results in failure for the dentist, the patient, and the technician. But Drs. Garber, Goldstein, and Feinman thoughtfully and precisely demonstrate a simple, scientifically sound placement procedure that will automatically ensure success. Their explanations are clear and will afford the dentist, the chairside dental assistant, and the dental technician a "blueprint" to thoroughly understand successful placement of laminate veneer restorations.

I particularly enjoyed the discussion of the various material alternatives for laminate veneer restorations, such as composite resin. The authors' prognostications on the future of laminate veneer technology and the direction that it may lead us in the future of esthetic dentistry is insightful and certainly stimulating.

I must take this singular opportunity to thank Drs. Garber, Goldstein, and Feinman for writing this excellent book about laminate veneers and its place in the field of esthetic dentistry, and for upholding the finest principles and ideals of the Academy of Esthetic Dentistry and its co-founder, Dr. Charles Pincus.

Frank R. Faunce, D.D.S.
Atlanta, Georgia

Acknowledgements

The very newness of the techique for laminating teeth with porcelain veneers indicates the enormous amount of time, effort, and research that must go in to bringing forth a text on the technique. We acknowledge the early efforts of Alain Rochette, Harold Horn, John Calamia, and Thomas Greggs during the neophyte stages of this process. Their innovative ideas and knowledge as well as the expertise of master ceramist Tokuo Masuda carried us through those early stages.

The artistry and skill of Pinhas Adar is evident throughout most of the chapters in this text. His creativity has been an integral part in creating the illusion of naturalness in porcelain laminates. His concept of P.A. opacity lends vitality to the laminates and has been so important in their acceptance as a cosmetic restoration.

We appreciate the efforts of all of the members of our office staff, particularly Kim Nimmons and Ginny Iwaniec, who spent many late evenings collating the materials we needed. Margie Smith has been a stalwart who has typed this manuscript at every odd hour of the day trying to meet continuous deadlines. Thanks also go to Chris Petree who put the text on a computer to simplify changing and rearranging as new information became available, and Denise Sabol who helped in so many ways.

The many colleagues who have been so supportive and helpful in the development of this concept need to be recognized: Frank Faunce, who kindly wrote the foreword to this text, and the enthusiastic efforts of Robert Nixon and Robert Ibsen, for their excellent work in promoting the concept of porcelain laminates. We would also like to recognize David Baird, Harry Albers, and especially Ron Jordan and Gordon Christensen for their help and support. We appreciate the support from our associates Brian Beaudreau, Cathy Schwartz, and Cary Goldstein. Howard Golden and John Johnny of Minolta have been a great source of photographic information.

No one pays more for our endeavors than our three families: wives, Barbara, Judy, and Billie, and our respective children, Karen, Jennifer, Michael, Rick, Ken, Jodi, Jill, and Dori.

Historical Perspectives

Thomas Greggs

Creating the perfect smile for Hollywood film actors in the 1930s was a significant part of Dr. Charles Pincus's California dental practice. The perfect mouth appearance necessary for motion pictures was certainly not a reality for the average person at that time. But the message Pincus delivered in his 1937 address before the California State Dental Association was poignant, stating that:

> The average dentist has a tendency to think only in terms of articulation and function with a little thought of esthetics thrown in for good measure. . . . We should always keep in mind that we are dealing with organs which can change an individual's entire visual personality. A captivating smile showing an even row of natural, gleaming white teeth is a major factor in achieving that elusive dominant characteristic known as personality.[1]

Pincus was fully aware of the importance of the "Hollywood smile" as an integral part of image, personality, and public opinion. Challenged by the need to develop an esthetic temporary restoration for those actors who did not want teeth cut down for full crowns, Pincus developed thin facings made of air-fired porcelain, which were temporarily held in place with adhesive denture powder while actors were before the camera. These facings presented a viable option to the full crown for actors who needed to temporarily change their smile, yet they possessed very little strength, and the technology necessary to provide a permanent means of attaching the veneers to tooth structure was lacking.

The art of veneering teeth has progressed over 30 years to the current generation of concepts and materials, which can be divided into two categories: *(1)* directly fabricated composite resin veneers (i.e., free-hand placed), and *(2)* indirectly fabricated veneers, such as preformed laminates or laboratory fabricated acrylic resin, microfill resin, or porcelain veneers.[2]

Direct Veneers

Buonocore's[3] research of the acid etch technique in 1955, combined with Bowen's[4,5] later use of filled resins, provided the technology enabling mechanical bonding between etched tooth and filled resins (direct bonding). Although these were major breakthroughs in dental research by the early 1960s, little esthetic use was made of this bonding technology for nearly a decade.[6] This was partially due to the limitations of the available self-curing resins, which did not allow sufficient working time for the dentist to re-create a labial surface before the composite resin chemically cured itself. Not until the 1970s did the practice of bonding composite resin directly to teeth for esthetic improvement grow in popularity.

The introduction of light-cured composite resins in the early to mid 1970s allowed the dentist greater flexibility. The advantages of visible light-cured composite resins, such as greater working time and improved chemistry, versus the self-cured composite resins, marked the entrée into the next generation of esthetic materials. Visible light-cured composite resins were replacing self-cured composite resins by the late 1970s and were preferred for esthetic anterior restorations.

Direct acid-etched bonding proved to be advantageous, yet a susceptibility to stain, poor wear resistance, and lack of natural fluorescence spurred the continued search for improved materials.[6–8]

Indirect Veneers

The idea of restoring teeth for esthetic purposes became more widely accepted by the dental community as new esthetic restorative techniques and materials became available. Faunce described a one-piece acrylic resin prefabricated veneer as an improved alternative to direct acid-etched bonding.[7,8] By using a chemical primer applied to the veneer and a composite resin to lute the veneer onto an etched tooth, both a chemical and mechanical bond contributed to the attachment. It was more stain resistant than composite resin veneers, but numerous preformed acrylic resin laminates suffered from delamination at the laminate/composite interface, usually due to the weak chemical bond.[9] Like composite resins, they also exhibited poor resistance to abrasion.

The inherent advantage to laboratory fabricated veneers is the anatomical accuracy created by the technician, thus alleviating the chairside artistry required with directly applied veneers. Laboratory formed acrylic resin veneers and laboratory formed microfill resin veneers offer a smooth surface, good masking ability, and very little finishing, if they are completed properly.[2] However, their esthetics, strength, and longevity can be surpassed by porcelain laminates.[10]

Porcelain Veneers

Glazed porcelain has a long history of use in dentistry as one of the most esthetic and biocompatible materials available, surpassed only by enamel itself.[6,11] Porcelain's abrasion and stain resistance are excellent and it is well tolerated by gingival tissues. The advent of porcelain labial veneers as a permanent esthetic restoration marked the progression of more than 30 years of dental research in acid-etch, bonding, and esthetic restorative techniques. The concept of acid etching porcelain was cited in the dental literature in 1975 when Rochette described the innovative restoration of a fractured incisor with an "etched silanted porcelain block."[11] In the early 1980s key pioneers in American laminate dentistry were instrumental in the development of porcelain veneers and the associated techniques for their fabrication and placement.[6,7,9,12–18]

Essential to the attachment of porcelain veneers is the ability of porcelain to be etched and bonded to composite resin and to exhibit a high tensile bond strength, as reported by Simonsen and Calamia.[15] Continued research by Calamia and Simonsen also showed that treatment of the etched porcelain veneer with a silane coupling agent produced a chemical bond that enhanced the porcelain/composite resin mechanical bond.[16]

The strength and durability of porcelain laminates will continue to be assessed. Although relatively technique-sensitive, the surface texture, color, fluorescence, and overall esthetics of porcelain laminate veneers have been regarded as exceptional.[2,6,9] In addition, the ability to adjust final color during placement allows maximum flexibility in final shade adjustment.

Esthetics in our culture has become a matter of necessary concern to the dentist. Changing trends and treatments for dental disease have made it necessary to diversify dental services.[17,18] It is predicted that the demand for esthetic dental services will continue to grow, prompted by an increasing population of consumers more knowledgeable in esthetic dental care options.[19,20]

When speaking of "mouth personality," Dr. Charles Pincus became aware of the actors' characters as he recreated their smiles to suit those personalities. Smiles that were once reserved for Hollywood are now accessible to all who choose to look their best, "smile, relax, and be themselves."[1]

References

1. Pincus, C.R. Building mouth personality. J. Calif. S. Dent. Assoc. 14:125−129, 1938.

2. Christiansen, G.J. Veneering of teeth. State of the art. Dent. Clin. North Am. 29(2):373−391, 1985.

3. Buonocore, M.G.A. Simple method of increasing the adhesion of acrylic filling materials to enamel surfaces. J. Dent. Res. 34:849−853, 1955.

4. Bowen, R.L. Development of a silica-resin direct filling material. Report 6333. Washington: National Bureau of Standards, 1958.

5. Bowen, R.L. Properties of a silica-reinforced polymer for dental restorations. J. Am. Dent. Assoc. 66: 57−64, 1963.

6. McLaughlin, G. Porcelain fused to tooth—a new esthetic and reconstructive modality. Compend. Cont. Educ. Dent. 5(5):430−435, 1985.

7. Faunce, F.R., and Myers, D.R. Laminate veneer restoration of permanent incisors. J. Am. Dent. Assoc. 93:790−792, 1976.

8. Faunce, F.R. Method and apparatus for restoring badly discolored, fractured or cariously involved teeth. United States Patent Number: 3,986,261. Filed Dec. 5, 1973. Date of Patent: Oct. 19, 1976.

9. Calamia, J.R. Etched porcelain veneers: the current state of the art. Quintessence Int. 16:5−12, 1985.

10. Comparison of Veneer Types. Clinical Research Associates Newsletter. Provo, Utah. 10(4), 1986.

11. Rochette, A. A ceramic restoration bonded by etched enamel and resin for fractured incisors. J. Prosthet. Dent. 33:287−293, 1975.

12. Boksman, L., et al. Etched porcelain labial veneers. Ont. Dent. 62(1):15−19, 1985.

13. Greggs, T.S. Method for cosmetic restoration of anterior teeth. United States Patent Number: 4,473,353. Filed April 15, 1983. Date of Patent: Sept. 25, 1984.

14. Horn, H.R. Porcelain laminate veneers bonded to etched enamel. Dent. Clin. North Am. 27:671−684, 1983.

15. Simonsen, R.J., and Calamia, J.R. Tensile bond strength of etched porcelain. J. Dent. Res.(Abstr. no. 1154), March, 1983.

16. Calamia, J.R., and Simonsen, R.J. Effect of coupling agents on bond strength of etched porcelain. J. Dent. Res. 63:162−362, 1984.

17. Goldstein, R.E. Communicating esthetics. N.Y. State Dent. J. 15(8):477−479, 1985.

18. Goldstein, R.E. Esthetics in Dentistry. Philadelphia: J.B. Lippincott, 1976.

19. Nixon, R. Personal communication, 1985.

20. Ibsen, R. Personal communication, 1985.

Features of Porcelain Laminate Veneers

2

Today's consumer publications, from *The Saturday Evening Post* through *Cosmopolitan, Town and Country,* and the *National Enquirer,* are replete with articles that emphasize the necessity and benefits of having beautiful teeth. The advent of bonding provided the concerned dentist with the means to attach composite resins, in their various shades, to the tooth surface in order to create esthetic illusions or to cover up unsightly teeth. A recent major breakthrough that facilitated predictable retention of porcelain to the tooth surface has added a new dimension to esthetic dentistry. Porcelain veneers can be considered to be very much the "state-of-the-art" in cosmetic dentistry because they offer innumerable advantages over any previous form of veneering systems.

Advantages of Porcelain Laminates

Porcelain as a replacement for unesthetic tooth substance has no peer for the following reasons:

- **Color.** This is a dual-fold advantage in that the porcelain offers better inherent color control and a natural look as well as the ongoing stability of these colors.
- **Bond strength.** The bond of the etched porcelain veneer to the enamel surface is considerably stronger than any other veneering system.
- **Periodontal health.** This highly glazed porcelain surface provides less of a depository area for plaque accumulation as compared to any other veneer system, and it appears that some types of porcelain veneers actually deter plaque accumulation.
- **Resistance to abrasion.** The wear and abrasion resistance is exceptionally high compared to composite resin.
- **Inherent porcelain strength.** The veneer itself is rather fragile, but once it is luted to enamel the restoration develops both high tensile and shear strengths. This is clinically evident by the fact that veneers cannot be "popped" off teeth but actually have to be ground away using rotary diamonds through to the original tooth surface. The cohesive strength of porcelain is considerably greater than the bond between resin particles and filler in a composite resin. Porcelain can therefore be used to increase the length of any given tooth by extending it over the incisal edge, both because the bond strength to enamel is so much higher and because the actual strength of the porcelain (i.e., adhesive and cohesive strengths) is greater.
- **Resistance to fluid absorption.** Porcelain absorbs fluids to a lesser degree than any other veneering material.
- **Esthetics.** The esthetics are considerably better than any other veneering material because of the ability to control color and surface texture with ceramic. Porcelain can be stained both internally and superficially and has a natural fluorescence, lending a certain vitality. Texture is readily developed on the veneer surface to simulate that of adjacent teeth and can be maintained indefinitely.

Disadvantages of Porcelain Laminates

- **Time.** The placing of veneers is technique sensitive and therefore time consuming.
- **Repair.** The veneers cannot be easily repaired once they are luted to the enamel.
- **Technique-sensitive.** The process of making veneers is an indirect one, requiring two patient visits, impression making, and laboratory fees.
- **Color.** It is difficult to modify color once the veneers are luted in position on the enamel surface.
- **Tooth preparation.** Some tooth preparation may be required to prevent potential problems associated with overcontouring.
- **Fragility.** The veneers are extremely fragile and difficult to manipulate.
- **Cost.** The dental fee for a porcelain laminate can generally range from three quarters of the fee to even more than the normal fee for an anterior full crown. This should depend on the difficulty of the patient's problem, the time, level of skill, artistic requirements, planning, and laboratory costs involved, and finally on whatever "guarantee" you decide to offer the patient regarding length of service and under what conditions you agree to replace or repair the laminate at no additional fee.

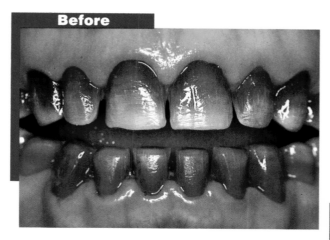

Fig. 2-1a Severe tetracycline stain coupled with small, multiple diastemata can be seen in this patient's smile.

Fig. 2-1b Maxillary porcelain laminates were placed extending to the first molars, and mandibular laminates were placed extending to the first premolars. Gross discoloration was neutralized by the "P" opacity in the laminates themselves.

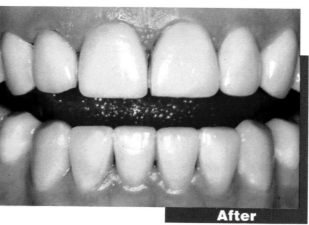

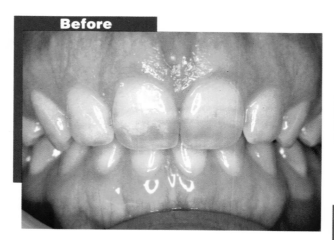

Fig. 2-2a This patient shows streaked discoloration of the enamel with lingually inclined teeth, postorthodontically.

Fig. 2-2b The discoloration has been entirely covered up, yet the shading remains natural and the lingual incline of the teeth has been compensated for by building the laminates out buccally.

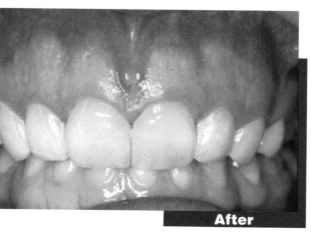

Fig. 2-3a This patient had a medium-sized diastema between the two central incisors, with a Class IV fracture of the left central incisor.

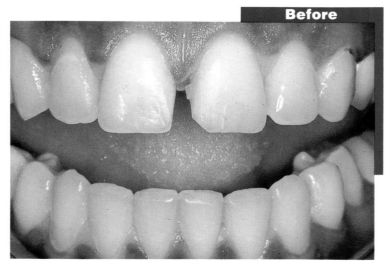

Before

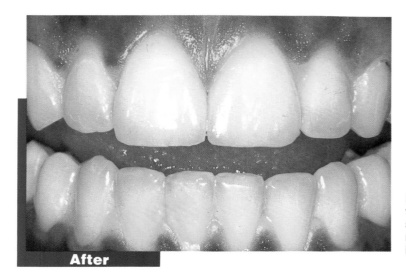

After

Fig. 2-3b Two labial veneers were placed to close the diastema and repair the fractured mesial corner of the left central incisor.

Indications

Dentistry has long sought the ideal restorative material to esthetically alter unattractive smiles. Although porcelain veneers are no panacea, they do offer solutions that are both conservative in nature and esthetically pleasing for the following clinical situations:

- **Discoloration.** Teeth discolored by tetracycline staining, devitalization, and fluorosis, and even teeth darkened with age can benefit by the process. Patients can be given younger, brighter-looking smiles (Figs. 2-1a and b).

- **Enamel defects.** Different types of enamel hypoplasia and malformations can be masked (Figs. 2-2a and b).
- **Diastemata.** Gaps (Figs. 2-3a and b) and other multiple unsightly spaces (Figs. 2-4a to d) can be closed.
- **Malpositioned teeth.** Developing the esthetic illusion of straight teeth where teeth are actually rotated or malpositioned can be accomplished for patients who have relatively sound teeth but do not wish to undergo orthodontics (Figs. 2-5a to f).

Fig. 2-4a Bleaching has lightened the teeth of this patient somewhat, but the teeth are still dark and there are multiple spaces between the anterior teeth.

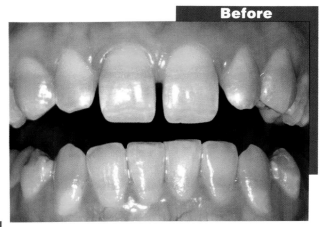

Fig. 2-4b Eight maxillary laminates were placed to compensate for the color and to close the spaces.

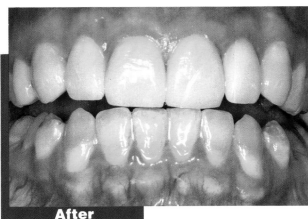

Fig. 2-4c The patient's smile before laminates.

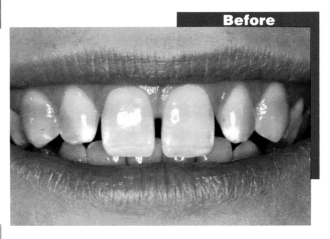

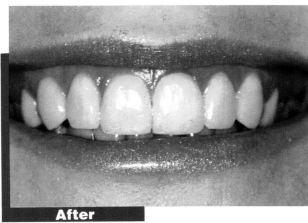

Fig. 2-4d The same smile following placement of eight laminates and mild shortening of the two central incisors.

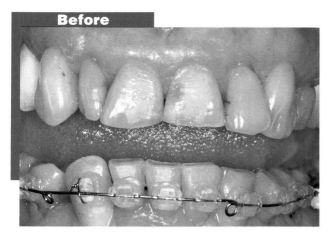

Before

Fig. 2-5a These malpositioned maxillary teeth show enamel hypoplasia and discoloration.

Fig. 2-5b Six laminates have been placed to compensate for the color and malposition of the teeth.

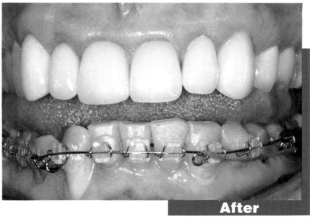

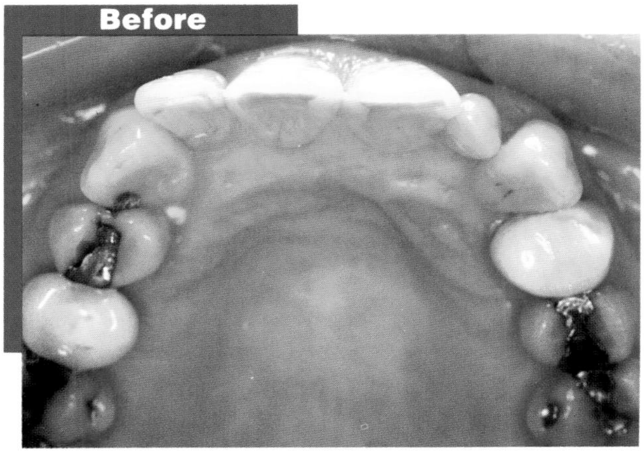

After

Fig. 2-5c The occlusal view shows poor anterior arch form with one labially placed lateral incisor and one rotated, lingually placed lateral incisor.

Fig. 2-5d The occlusal view now shows a well-rounded arch; the laminates have compensated for the poor position of the teeth.

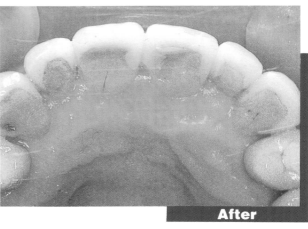

After

- **Malocclusion.** The configuration of lingual surfaces of anterior teeth can be changed to develop increased guidance or centric holding areas in malocclusions or periodontally compromised teeth.

- **Poor restorations.** Teeth with numerous, shallow, unesthetic restorations on labial surfaces can be dramatically restored.

- **Aging.** The ongoing process of aging can result in color changes and wear in teeth. This is often considered unesthetic to our youth- and beauty-orientated society. These teeth may be ideal candidates for improvement by bleaching or, in certain situations, bleaching with subsequent veneering (Figs. 2-6a and b).

- **Wear patterns.** Porcelain laminates are also useful in those cases that exhibit slowly progressive wear patterns. If sufficient enamel remains and the desired increase in length is not excessive, porcelain veneers can be bonded to the remaining tooth structure to change shape, color, or function (Figs. 2-7a and b).

- **Agenesis of the lateral incisor.** In the problem of the canine erupting adjacent to the central incisor (in those situations where there is a missing lateral incisor) the veneer can be used to develop better coronal form in the canine, thus simulating a lateral incisor. These may have to be combined with veneers on the central incisors to develop a more ideal ratio in the relative proportion of the teeth, because the canine is invariably too wide when positioned adjacent to the central incisor (Figs. 2-8a and b).

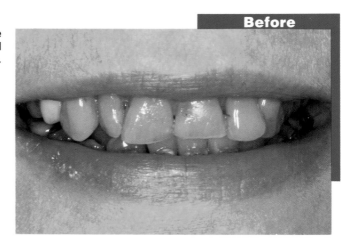

Fig. 2-5e Preoperative smile showing discolored, rotated teeth.

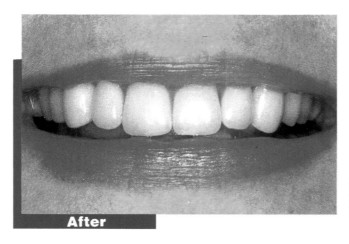

Fig. 2-5f The smile following placement of six laminates and four crowns on the premolars.

Fig. 2-6a Anterior teeth showing wear and some discoloration associated with the age of the patient.

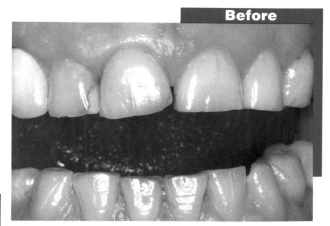
Before

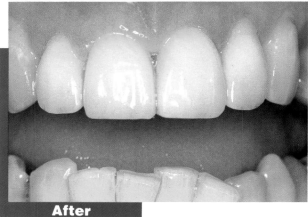
After

Fig. 2-6b Four laminates were placed to compensate for the discoloration and wear, but the natural look of the patient has been retained by a slight diastema between the two central incisors, the same labial position of the right lateral incisor, and mesial tilt to the right central incisor. This patient wanted to look younger than she had at presentation but did not want a typically "juvenile" white smile.

Fig. 2-7a Preoperative view showing some degree of wear on the right central incisor and severe wear on the lateral incisors.

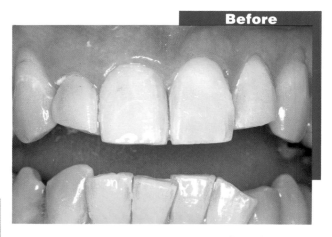
Before

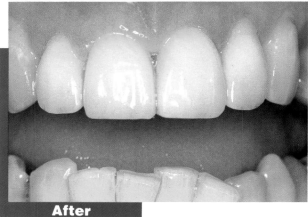
After

Fig. 2-7b Four laminates were placed following occlusal modification to develop guidance on the canines as opposed to the lateral incisors.

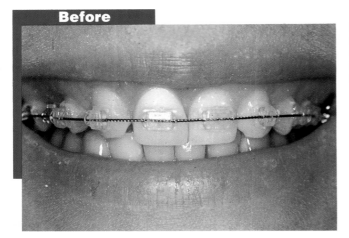

Before

Fig. 2-8a This patient had missing lateral incisors and the canines were moved orthodontically immediately adjacent to the central incisors.

Fig. 2-8b Three conventional porcelain laminates and one Dicor (Dentsply/York Div., York, Pa.) crown on the maxillary right central incisor were placed to modify the coronal form on the canines and to simulate lateral incisors, whereas the central incisors were increased in size slightly to compensate for the large size of the canines.

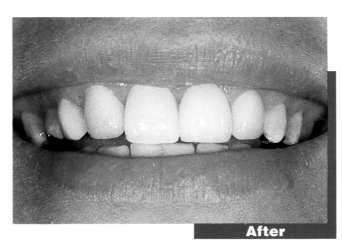

After

Summary of Porcelain Laminate Advantages and Disadvantages

Advantages	Disadvantages
• Color	• Time involved
• Bond strength	• Repair
• Periodontal health	• Technique-sensitive
• Resistance to abrasion	• Color
• Inherent porcelain strength	• Tooth preparation
• Resistance to fluid absorption	• Fragility
• Esthetics	• Cost

Contraindications

The authors do not consider there to be any specific contraindications for laminate veneers as opposed to other forms of dental restoration. There are, however, certain considerations to be taken into account:

- **Available enamel.** There should be enamel around the whole periphery of the laminate, not only for adhesion but, more importantly, to seal the veneer to the tooth surface. In addition there should be sufficient enamel available for bonding, because bonding to dentin is generally much less retentive than to enamel. If the tooth or teeth are composed predominantly of dentin and cementum, crowning may well be the treatment of choice.

- **Ability to etch enamel.** Deciduous teeth and teeth that have been excessively fluoridated may not etch effectively. They may require special measures to be successful with porcelain laminates.

- **Oral habits.** Patients with certain tooth-to-tooth habit patterns, such as bruxism, or tooth-to-foreign-objects habits may not be ideal candidates for veneers. The shearing stress may be too great for the porcelain to withstand.

The system's inherent strength and long-term stability indicate that there are few contraindications to porcelain laminate use, provided discretion is used in case selection and care is exercised in the preparation, fabrication, and placement of veneers.

Bibliography

Albers, H.F. Tooth Colored Restoratives. 7th ed. Cotati, Calif.: Alto Books, 1985.

Christensen, G.J. Comparison of veneer types. Clinical Research Associates Newsletter. Provo, Utah. 10(4):1–2, 1986.

Feinman, R.A. A combination therapy. Calif. Dent. Assoc. J. 15(4):10–13, 1987.

Fenton, S. Expert picks the ten best celebrity smiles. National Enquirer 60(51):17, July 22, 1986.

Freidman, M. Personal communication, 1985.

Goldstein, R.E. Diagnostic dilemma: to bond, laminate, or crown? Int. J. Periodont. Rest. Dent. 7(5):9–29, 1987.

Jordan, R.E. Esthetic Composite Bonding. Toronto, Philadelphia: B.C. Decker, 1986.

Murrell, G.A. Flash that smile. Shape Magazine 6(3):37–38, November 1986.

Nixon, R.L. The Chairside Manual for Porcelain Bonding. Wilmington, Del.: B.A. Videographics, 1987.

Wilson, J. Coming up smiling. Town & Country November 1985, pp. 220–295.

Wilson, J. I had a dental makeover. Cosmopolitan Magazine April 1987, pp. 170–172.

Dental Porcelain Technology

Dan Nathanson

Dental porcelain has become the most widely used material for the construction of crowns in dentistry because of its excellent esthetic properties and its ability to closely duplicate the appearance of natural tooth structure. The crystalline structure of porcelain gives it optical refractive properties similar to those of translucent enamel. Glazed porcelain surfaces, because they are smooth in texture and quite resistant to wear and discoloration, are durable.

But although processed dental porcelain has a high compressive strength, it is completely nonductile and therefore brittle. Also, because of surface irregularities inherent in the manufacturing process, dental porcelain restorations have a low tensile strength. *These surface irregularities, even though microscopic in size, can cause significant stress concentration.* In the nonductile porcelain, stresses cannot be relieved by plastic deformation (as is possible in metals) and even minor defects under tensile stresses may develop into larger cracks by a mechanism of crack propagation. Ultimately, the process may cause ad-

ditional stress concentration and failure in the form of a brittle fracture.[1]

Methods of Strengthening Porcelain

Because of the inherent weakness of dental porcelain, different methods to strengthening it have been developed. The porcelain-fused-to-metal restoration is probably the most well-known example for a porcelain strengthening system and allows porcelain to be effectively used in dental restorations. The metal structure provides, in addition to accurate fit, a mechanism to prevent porcelain failure under tensile stresses. Other commonly used porcelain reinforcing methods are metallic foil substructures,[2] the aluminous porcelain core, and the more recently introduced magnesia-alumina spinel.[3]

24

Etched Porcelain

The porcelain restoration as presented in this book makes use of a substantially different concept for the reinforcement of the brittle ceramic. This new treatment modality employs the fine etching of the porcelain inner surface both for retention and porcelain reinforcement. The bonding resin used for "cementing" the porcelain restorations in place flows into the microdefects of the etched enamel on the tooth side and the etched porcelain on the restoration side, bonding the two together. The polymerized resin provides considerable retention and simultaneously protects the porcelain from cracking and fracturing under tensile stresses. This is similar to the strengthening effect of the metal in the porcelain-fused-to-metal restoration. With resin bonding of etched porcelain to tooth, part of the clinical success can be explained by the polymerization shrinkage of the resin (a property inherent in most polymers) which stresses the thin porcelain in a direction that reduces the chance of crack formation and propagation.

Fig. 3-1 SEM micrograph (original magnification × 1,000) of unetched porcelain surface.

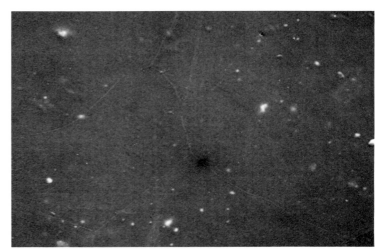

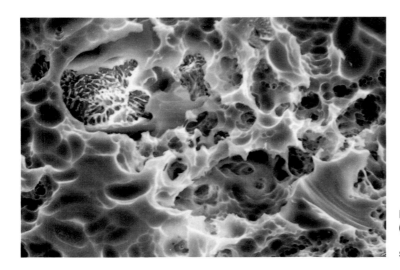

Fig. 3-2 SEM micrograph (original magnification × 1,000) of etched porcelain surface.

The retentive qualities of the porcelain surface may well depend upon the nature of the microscopic pattern produced during the etching process. Porcelain processed on a platinum foil exhibits a relatively smooth surface even under high magnification (Fig. 3-1). Etching the porcelain surface with hydrofluoric acid (or a derivative) produces the microscopic surface roughness (Fig. 3-2) that provides retention when combined with a flowing resin capable of polymerizing. Early etching methods for porcelain consisted of either a 15-minute etch with a 10% hydrofluoric acid or a 20-minute etch with a commercial preparation consisting primarily of diluted hydrofluoric acid.[4] Initial bond strength values based on these etching methods[5] were reported to be around 1,100 psi. These values, although of clinical significance, were relatively low compared to bond values for resin to etched enamel, which were generally reported to be within 1,700 psi.[6]

The Effects of Solution and Time on Etching

A more recent look at etching patterns produced by various porcelain processing methods and different etching regimens produced interesting information in regard to the effect of etching solution and etching time. In an in vitro experiment,[7] flat, round porcelain samples (Microbond, Austenal Dental, Chicago, Ill.) were processed by the manufacturer either on platinum foil or a refractory bed. All porcelain samples were divided into groups for a variety of etching treatments as follows: (1) etching with hydrofluoric acid for 1.5 minutes, and (2) etching with Stripit (Keystone, Philadelphia, Pa.) for 1, 2.5, 5, 10, 15, and 20 minutes. The dried etched surfaces were examined in a scanning electron microscope and revealed different etching patterns (Figs. 3-3 to 3-8). A close examination of the patterns resulted in the selection of the refractory processed porcelain treated for 2.5 minutes of etching with Stripit solution as the most retentive pattern, because of its morphology.

This retentive etching pattern was tested for resin-to-porcelain bond strength by Hsu et al.[7] in an experiment of four groups, as shown in Table 3-1. A composite resin was bonded to all porcelain samples in this experiment by filling small, cylindrical celluloid capsules with a powder-liquid com-

Table 3-1 List of experimental groups

Group	Porcelain surface	Bonding promoter
1	Unetched	None
2	Unetched	Silane
3	Etched	None
4	Etched	Silane

posite resin (Ultra Bond, Den-Mat Corp., Santa Maria, Calif.) and positioning these capsules over the porcelain flat surfaces. The composite resin samples were light activated, and after aging for seven days in water they were tested for shear bond strength in a testing machine (Fig. 3-9). The results are shown in Fig. 3-10.

A comparison of the four groups revealed the effect of the silane bonding agent versus that of the etched porcelain. It is clear from this experiment that etching the porcelain is the predominant factor in producing the retention. But the combination of porcelain etching with a silane bonding promoter seems to have a cumulative effect that maximizes the bond strength significantly. The value of 3,500 psi for the group combining porcelain etching and silane pretreatment is far better than bond strengths obtained in early experiments. This bond also surpasses the resin-enamel bond strength.

An analysis of the etched porcelain/resin interface by means of scanning electron microscopy produced interesting information. In the nonetched porcelain groups a gap existed between the porcelain and resin that was most probably produced by the polymerization contraction of the resin (Fig. 3-11). The silane treatment caused a narrowing of the gap, apparently as a result of improved chemical attraction (Fig. 3-12).

In the etched porcelain, silane-treated groups no gap was found (Fig. 3-13), and the resin seemed to have filled all the porcelain defects. Apparently, the rough etched surface treated with silane produced a surface attraction, causing the resin to wet it well. The good adaptation of resin to etched porcelain seems to have produced the highest bond strengths.

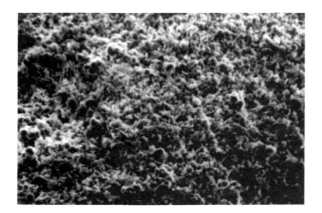

Fig. 3-3 SEM micrograph (original magnification × 500) of porcelain fired on investment and etched with hydrofluoric acid for 90 seconds.

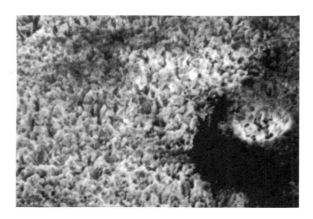

Fig. 3-4 SEM micrograph (original magnification × 500) of porcelain fired on platinum foil, etched with hydrofluoric acid for 90 seconds.

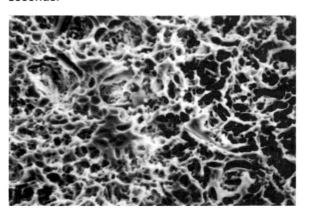

Fig. 3-5 SEM micrograph (original magnification × 500) of porcelain fired on investment, etched with diluted hydrofluoric acid for 2.5 minutes.

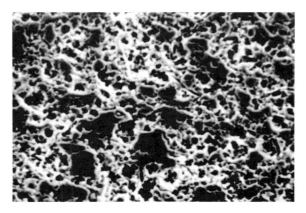

Fig. 3-6 SEM micrograph (original magnification × 500) of porcelain fired on platinum foil, etched with diluted hydrofluoric acid for 2.5 minutes.

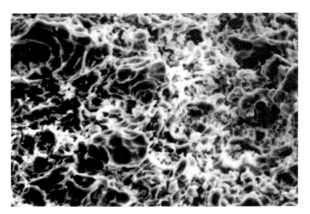

Fig. 3-7 SEM micrograph (original magnification × 500) of porcelain fired on investment, etched with diluted hydrofluoric acid for five minutes.

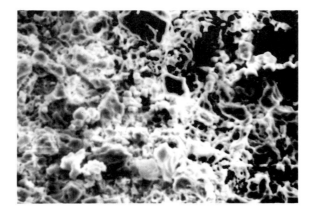

Fig. 3-8 SEM micrograph (original magnification × 500) of porcelain fired on platinum foil, etched with diluted hydrofluoric acid for 20 minutes.

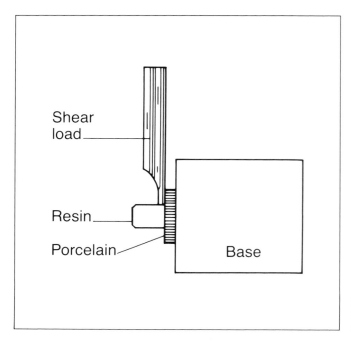

Fig. 3-9 Schematic representation of resin-porcelain bond strength testing.

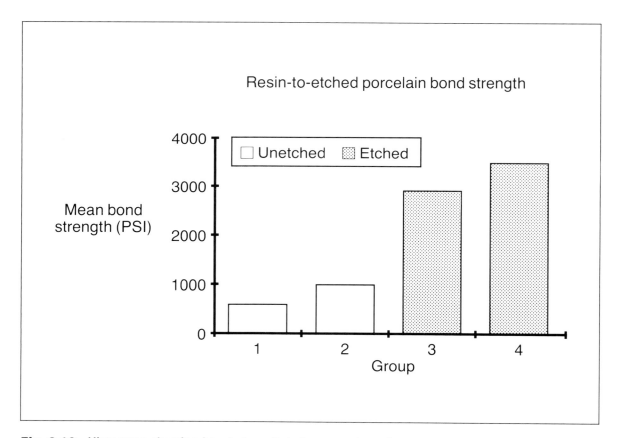

Fig. 3-10 Histogram showing bond strength between resin and porcelain samples treated as described in Table 3-1.

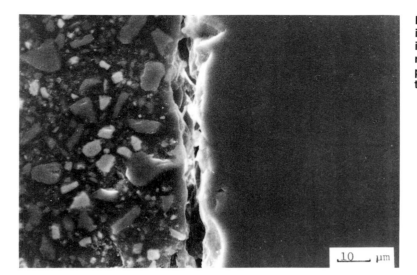

Fig. 3-11 SEM micrograph (original magnification × 1,000) showing interface between composite resin and unetched, untreated porcelain. Note gap between the two materials.

Fig. 3-12 Interface between composite resin and unetched porcelain treated with silane (SEM, original magnification × 1,000). Note narrowing of gap as compared to Fig. 3-11.

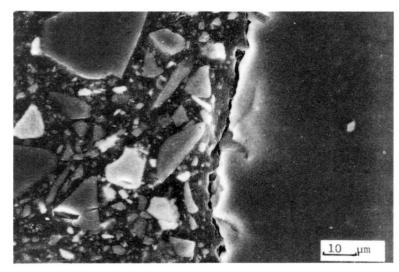

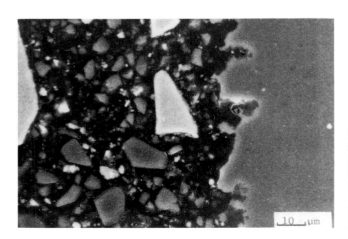

Fig. 3-13 Interface between composite resin and etched porcelain treated with silane and a dentin bonding agent (SEM, original magnification × 1,000). No gap is noted—the resin fills all porcelain surface irregularities.

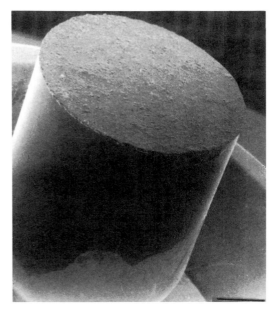

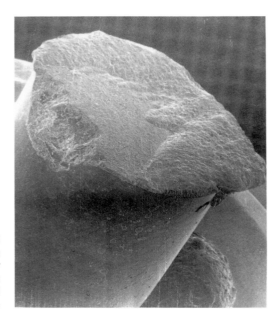

Fig. 3-14 SEM micrograph (original magnification × 20) of separated resin cylinder from unetched group after shear testing. Clean top surface suggests adhesive failure.

Fig. 3-15 SEM micrograph (original magnification × 20) of separated resin cylinder from etched porcelain after shear testing. A portion of the porcelain substrate fractured and remained adhered to the resin sample.

Low magnification SEM analysis of the resin cylinders after their separation from the etched porcelain surfaces revealed different failure mechanisms for the various groups. Nonetched porcelain produced an adhesive failure between the resin and the porcelain, and the flat resin surface remained unaffected (Fig. 3-14). In the etched porcelain groups, adhesive failures within the porcelain structure occurred as evidenced by porcelain pieces that remained bonded to the composite resin cylinder after separation (Fig. 3-15).

Both the silane and the etched porcelain surface contribute to the retention of the resin. Silane use for enhancing the bond between porcelain and acrylic resin has been reported by Semmelman and Kulp[8] and Paffenbarger et al.[9] Myerson reported better bonds with cold-cured versus heat-cured acrylic when using silane.[10] Newbury and Pameijer[11] used silane in bonding a porcelain tooth with composite resin. The study by Hsu et al.[7] established that *the etching of the porcelain is the cardinal element in obtaining good retention* with the resin, but the effect of the silane coupler is also measurable and is cumulative with that of the etching. Thus, the combined etching and silane treatment produced the highest bond strength.

In a continuation of the Hsu et al. bond strength experiment, Nathanson et al.[12] kept samples from all four groups in water at room temperature for 6 months and 30 months and then subjected them to a shear load. This test was undertaken to measure the long-term effect of exposure to water and possible hydration of the resins and bonding components in the system. Mean bond strengths for the four experimental groups at 6 months and 30 months along with the original results are presented in Table 3-2. Figure 3-16 is a graphic representation of the immediate and long-term bond strength date. The results show a general trend toward reductions of bond strengths with time exposure. However, the silane-treated etched porcelain showed a relatively small change and maintained a mean bond strength of 3,000 to 3,150 psi over the 30-month period.

In another experiment, the effect of the addition of a dental bonding agent was also tested and compared to groups bonded with silane.[13] With unetched porcelain, the dental bonding agent significantly improved the resin-to-porcelain bond strength. With etched porcelain, use of the dental bonding enhanced the bond strength, but the additional increment was not statistically significant. Still, *the use of a dental bonding agent in combination with etched porcelain is now recommended routinely.*

Table 3-2   Mean resin-to-etched porcelain bond strength after time exposure (psi)

	Time in water		
Group	7 days	6 months	30 months
1	564	390	468
2	978	693	567
3	2907	2191	2361
4	3485	2936	3170

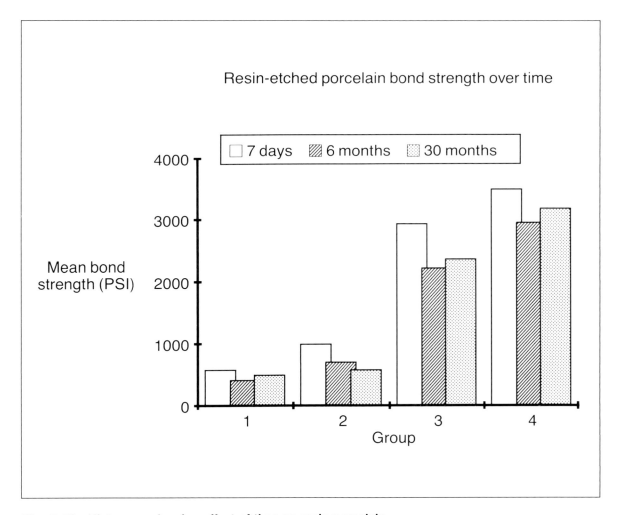

Fig. 3-16   Histogram showing effect of time on resin-porcelain bond strength in experimental groups described in Table 3-1.

Polymerization

Complete polymerization of the composite resin is another essential requirement for obtaining a good bond between the tooth and porcelain. Polymerization of light-activated composite resins is dependent on the transmission of light and its penetration through the porcelain into the composite resin. Several factors can affect this light transmission, but most important are the thickness of the porcelain and its opacity, and the opacity of the composite resin used. An in vitro study by Nathanson and Hassan employed porcelain tablets of different thickness ranging from 1.4 to 4.6 mm.[14] These porcelain samples were etched on one surface. Celluloid cylinders filled with a light-curing composite resin were positioned over the etched surfaces, but the curing light was transmitted through the porcelain by using a special jig (Fig. 3-17). Several resin bonding systems were tested (Table 3-3). The results as shown in Fig. 3-18 indicate that resin-to-porcelain bond strength is indeed a function of porcelain thickness: the thicker the porcelain, the lower the bond strength. Systems with a dual polymerization initiation system (photo *and* chemical curing) give a significantly better bond strength with thick porcelain than do systems that polymerize solely by light. Visible light polymerization shows a sub-stantial reduction in effectiveness when the light has to travel through more than 3 mm of porcelain.

The subject of resin polymerization is extremely important because retention and mechanical support to the brittle porcelain restorations are a direct function of the degree of polymerization. Incomplete polymerization reduces bond strength significantly, as evidenced in the in vitro experiment,[14] and may contribute to early clinical separation and failure. The phenomenon of incomplete polymerization is more likely to occur in thick etched porcelain restorations, such as inlays or onlays, where the thickness of porcelain may approach 4 to 8 mm in some areas. In the thin anterior porcelain veneers, this is less likely to occur because the light can easily penetrate through 0.5 to 1 mm of porcelain. However, in interproximal regions where the light rays might enter at an angle to the porcelain surface, the degree of penetration and degree of polymerization may be reduced. In both thin and thick etched porcelain restorations, *immediate retention* will not be affected because some thin sections probably exist that will allow full setting of the resin in those sections. ***The restoration will therefore appear secure in place, but it may contain much unreacted resin that could eventually wash out and cause marginal caries.***

Table 3-3 **Resin-porcelain bond strength (psi) versus porcelain thickness***

Group	Material	1.4 mm		4.6 mm	
		Mean	S.D.	Mean	S.D.
A	Ultra Bond†	2304	248	1568	⌈ 208
E	Marathon† (dual cure)	1927	84	1525	⌊ 155
C	Durafill‡	1464	84	920	72
B	Porcelite§	1865	204	342	62
D	Marathon†	1385	84	84	22

*Values within bracket not significantly different.
†Den-Mat Corp., Santa Maria, Calif.
‡Kulzer, Inc., Irvine, Calif.
§Kerr/Sybron, Romulus, Mich.

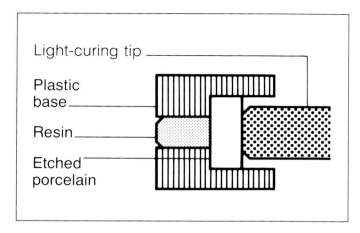

Fig. 3-17 Schematic representation of a laboratory experiment to test effect of light transmission through porcelain on curing of composite resin.

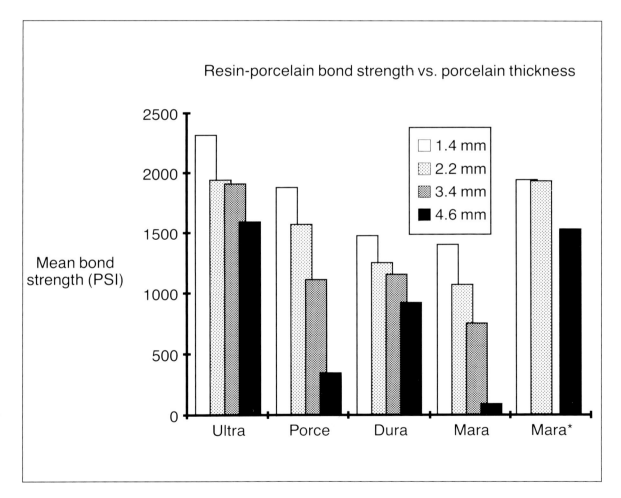

Resin-porcelain bond strength vs. porcelain thickness

Fig. 3-18 Histogram showing effect of porcelain thickness on resin-porcelain bond strength. *ULTRA* (Ultra Bond, Dent-Mat Corp., Santa Maria, Calif.); *PORCE* (Porcelite, Kerr/Sybron, Romulus, Mich.); *DURA* (Durafill, Kulzer, Inc., Irvine, Calif.); *MARA* (Marathon, Den-Mat Corp.); *MARA** (Dual Cure Marathon, Den-Mat Corp.).

Longevity of Porcelain Restorations

Etched porcelain restorations are not subject to surface wear, roughness, or discoloration, as may be the case with some direct composite resins. However, longevity of these restorations is dependent primarily on the bond strength between the restoration and the underlying dental tissue.[15] A weak resin-to-porcelain bond (or deterioration of the bond with time) will cause early failure of the restoration by subjecting it to the possibility of deformation and fracture.

In clinical usage, therefore, obtaining an optimal porcelain-to-resin bond strength is of utmost importance for durability.

Longevity of a restoration cannot be predicted merely by testing its mechanical properties in vitro, and only clinical data may provide the answer. With anterior etched porcelain restorations, the longest clinical experience reported to date has been from three to eight years.[16, 17] Still, based on clinical experience with direct bonding and the knowledge of resin and porcelain properties, it is likely that the etched porcelain restorations will last as long as (if not longer than) porcelain crowns. In certain aspects, such as the preservation of more tooth structure and the elimination of a soluble cement, the etched porcelain restorations may well be superior to the conventionally used ceramic crowns.

References

1. Phillips, R.W. Science of Dental Materials. 8th ed. Philadelphia: W.B. Saunders Co., 1982, p. 510.

2. McLean, J.W., and Sced, I.R. The bonded alumina crown. I. The bonding of platinum to aluminous dental porcelain using tin-oxide coatings. Aust. Dent. J. 21:119, 1976.

3. Starling, L.B., Stephan, J.E., and Stroud, R.D. Shrink-free ceramic and method and raw batch for the manufacture thereof. United States Patent Number 4,265,669. 1981.

4. Horn, H.R. Porcelain laminate veneers bonded to etched enamel. Dent. Clin. North Am. 27:671, 1983.

5. Simonsen, R.J., and Calamia, J.R. Tensile bond strength of etched porcelain. J. Dent. Res. 62(Spec. Issue; Abstr. no. 1154), 1983.

6. Fusayama, T. New Concepts in Operative Dentistry. Chicago: Quintessence Publ. Co., 1980, p. 69.

7. Hsu, C.S., Stangel, I., and Nathanson, D. Shear bond strength of resin to etched porcelain. J. Dent. Res. 64(Spec. Issue; Abstr. no. 1095):269, 1985.

8. Semmelman, J.O., and Kulp, P.R. Silane bonding porcelain teeth to acrylic. J. Am. Dent. Assoc. 76:69, 1968.

9. Paffenbarger, G.C., Sweeney, W.T., and Bowers, R.L. Bonding porcelain teeth to acrylic resin denture bases. J. Am. Dent. Assoc. 74:1018, 1967.

10. Myerson, R.L. Effects of silane bonding of acrylic resins to porcelain on porcelain structure. J. Am. Dent. Assoc. 78:113, 1969.

11. Newburg, R., and Pameijer, C.H. Composite resins bonded to porcelain with silane solution. J. Am. Dent. Assoc. 96:288, 1978.

12. Nathanson, D., Stangel, I., and Hsu, C.S. Effect of time on resin to etched porcelain bond strength. (Unpublished data.)

13. Stangel, I., Nathanson, D., and Hsu, C.S. Shear strength of composite bonded to etched porcelain. J. Dent. Res. (In press.)

14. Nathanson, D., and Hassan F. Effect of etched porcelain thickness on resin-porcelain bond strength. J. Dent. Res. 66(Spec. Issue; Abstr. no. 1107), 1987.

15. Nathanson, D. Etched porcelain restorations for improved esthetics. I. Anterior veneers. Compend. Cont. Educ. Dent. 7:706, 1986.

16. Calamia, J.R., et al. Clinical evaluation of etched porcelain laminate veneers: results at (6 months–3 years). J. Dent. Res. 66(Spec. Issue; Abstr. no. 1110), 1987.

17. Jenkins, C.B.G., and Aboush, Y.E.Y. Clinical durability of porcelain laminates over 8 years. J. Dent. Res. 60:1081, 1987.

Enamel Reduction

4

There are different opinions regarding the type of tooth preparation porcelain laminate veneers require. Some clinicians are of the school of thought that little or no tooth reduction is required, whereas others, at the opposite end of the spectrum, advocate a full, deep chamfer preparation on the labial aspect of the teeth and most or all of the way through the interproximal contact areas.

There is as yet no scientific data available to support either school of thought, and it is the opinion of the authors that both concepts may be correct or incorrect. With each specific case in hand, just how to approach the preparation should be decided on an individual basis. The philosophy presented in this book will be biologically based to produce an effective restoration with decreased potential for causing iatrogenic disease. If it is possible to place a veneer without tooth preparation and still develop good esthetic form with no subsequent periodontal changes, then this is obviously the ideal. If not, some form of enamel reduction becomes essential.

There is therefore no single answer or ideal way to prepare teeth for porcelain laminates. The decision of whether to reduce enamel should depend on the following biological and technical factors:

- **Esthetics.** If there is no tooth preparation, somewhat larger teeth more labially positioned will result when laminates are placed. In lingually inclined teeth this may be an advantage because the end result will correct the relative position of the teeth and be esthetically more pleasing.
- **Relative tooth position.** If one or more of the teeth are out of line with respect to the others, this will influence the degree of preparation necessary.
- **Masking of tetracycline stain.** This complex problem requires very specific preparation modifications.
- **Marginal placement.** This should be considered relative to the gingival margin.

- **Age.** The age of the patient and the proximity of the pulp to the surface needs to be taken into account.

- **Psyche.** The attitudes of the patient relative to esthetics in general, and tooth reduction in particular, should be determined prior to case presentation since this could modify the expected esthetic result.

- **The potential for periodontal changes.** The individual patient's past periodontal history and tissue susceptibility to bacterial plaque should be reviewed.

- **Plaque removal.** The patient should be evaluated for the ability to remove plaque at a porcelain/tooth interface.

If these restorations are to be esthetic and biologically compatible, they will often necessitate adjustment of the tooth surface. This reduction in enamel can then be replaced with a similar thickness of porcelain, thereby making the end result the same size or, at worst, only nominally larger than the original.

It is extremely difficult for the ceramist to fabricate an accurately fitting laminate to a feather edge finish line, or to work with a thickness much less than 0.3 mm. In broad generalities, then, the amount of enamel reduction necessary, based on the technician's needs, is in the realm of 0.3 to 0.6 mm or about half the thickness of the available enamel.

Enamel reduction should be considered from five distinct aspects:

- Labial reduction
- Interproximal extension
- Sulcular extension
- Incisal or occlusal modification
- Lingual reduction

Rationale for Enamel Preparation

Enamel preparation may be performed for several reasons:

- To provide for an adequate dimension of available space for the porcelain material

- To remove convexities and provide for a path of insertion in those situations where either the incisal or the interproximal areas are to be included in the veneer; the best path of insertion is that which will require the least amount of enamel reduction, as modified by esthetic demands of the patient

- To provide space for adequate opaquing where necessary and for the composite resin luting agent

- To provide a definite seat to help position the laminate during placement

- To prepare a receptive enamel surface for etching and bonding the laminate

- To facilitate sulcular margin placement in severely discolored teeth

---

Enamel Reduction Procedure

1. Labial Reduction

The labial preparation should encompass the amount of reduction necessary to facilitate the placement of an esthetic restoration. Ideally, one would like to replace the same amount of enamel that is removed by the preparation. However, in certain situations, such as rotated teeth or teeth in labial-version, it may be advantageous to first bring the offending teeth into alignment with the rest of the arch by reducing their labial contour.

The preparation should remain within the enamel wherever possible and most certainly at all the peripheral marginal areas to ensure an adequate seal to enamel.

There may be situations where in small areas, to facilitate cosmetic alignment, some amount of dentin will be exposed by the preparation of the tooth. This is not that critical if it is limited to only small areas and the margins remain on enamel. Dental bonding, however, provides only a fraction of the bond strength possible with enamel bond-

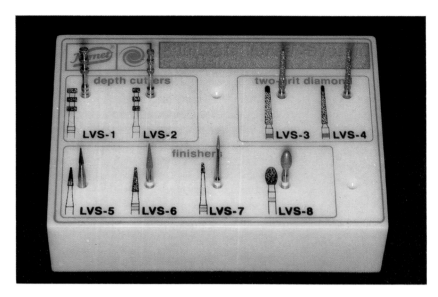

Fig. 4-1 The Brassler LVS Porcelain Laminate Preparation and Finishing Kit.

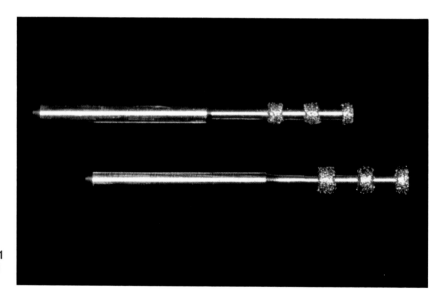

Fig. 4-2 The LVS nos. 1 and 2 depth cutters—0.3 and 0.5 mm.

ing and a less effective seal. ***Therefore, a good general rule may well be to ensure that over 50% of the preparation is on enamel.***

A problem with fresh dentin exposure is the potential of the acidic etching solution and the bonding material itself to cause pulpal hyperemia or even necrosis.

Depth Guide

To randomly grind away the enamel with no guideline of how much is being removed would be inappropriate. There are several methods to gauge the amount of enamel removed, one of the most effective being the LVS depth cutter diamond (Brasseler, Savannah, Ga.) (Fig. 4-1). This diamond stone will create horizontal striations or depth-cut grooves on the labial aspect of the tooth. The depth of the cut is limited by the shank which comes to rest on the surface of the uncut enamel between the striations (Fig. 4-5).

The depth-cutting diamond comes in two sizes (LVS no. 1 and LVS no. 2), one of which would be appropriate for the tooth to be prepared (Fig. 4-2). These dimensions are 0.5 mm reduction for most situations and 0.3 mm for small teeth such as mandibular incisors where the thickness of enamel is considerably less.

Make a decision on the required amount of reduction, then select the appropriate diamond depth cutter. Gently draw the diamond across the labial surface of the tooth in a mesial to distal direction. This will develop the depth cuts as horizontal grooves, leaving a raised strip of enamel between (Fig. 4-6).

Then remove this remaining enamel to the depth of the original grooves, thereby reducing the tooth the exact amount—no less and no more (Fig. 4-7). (There are some schools of thought that advocate leaving a degree of striation present as a definitive locating system for the laminate placement.)

In an alternative method for gauging the amount of enamel reduction that is somewhat more complex, use a no. 1 round bur. The depth from the peripheral aspect of the bur to the shank is 0.4 mm. Hold the bur at a slight angle so that indentations can be made into the enamel to the depth limited by the base of the shank. Create these indentations randomly across the surface of the enamel, thereby ensuring that subsequent reduction to the depth of these indentations will create a uniformly equal preparation on the labial aspect of the tooth. In addition, scribe a groove of the same depth following the curvature of the gingival margin. The problems with this type of approach are that these depth cuts can vary, depending on the angle the bur is held at, and that the amount of time necessary for this process is considerably greater.

Reduction of the Remaining Enamel

Following the creation of the depth cut or striations, the remaining enamel must be reduced to the depth of these initial cuts (Fig. 4-7). The labial reduction should encompass two aspects: (1) the bulk of the reduction should be done with a coarse

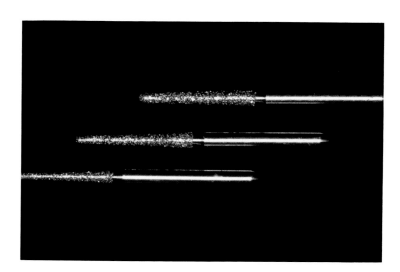

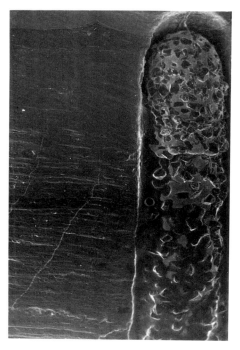

Fig. 4-3 *(above)* **The LVS nos. 3 and 4 two-grit diamond in a selection of three different sizes for different clinical situations.**

Fig. 4-4 *(right)* **Scanning electron microscope of an LVS two-grit diamond and the varying effects of the grit sizes on prepared enamel.**

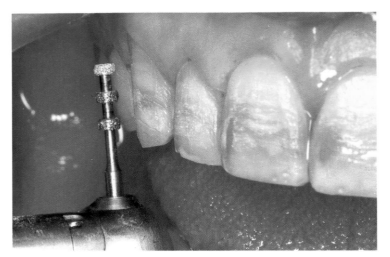

Fig. 4-5 Position the depth cutter on the labial aspect of the tooth to be prepared.

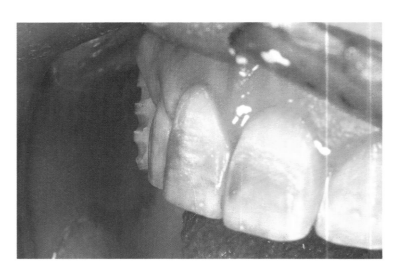

Fig. 4-6 Oblique view showing the 0.5-mm striations cut into the enamel by the depth cutter.

Fig. 4-7 Place the two-grit diamond into position and prepare the interspersed enamel down to the depth of the striations.

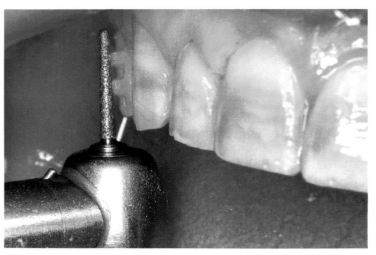

diamond in order to facilitate added retention and better refraction of the light being transmitted back out through the laminate, and *(2)* at the marginal area, it is desirable to use a fine-grit diamond that will create a definitive, smooth finish line to enhance the seal at the periphery.

The unique LVS two-grit diamond (Brasseler, Savannah, Ga.) (Fig. 4-3) is specifically designed to do this simultaneously with only one bur. It will rapidly remove coronal enamel with a coarse grit while creating the desired form of finish line with a fine diamond grit. This "two-grit" diamond concept is predicated upon these basic tenets of having a fine, polished finish line and a more coarsely prepared axial wall (Fig. 4-4). The instrument therefore has 1.3 mm of fine-grit diamond at the tip and a hybrid mixture of rapidly cutting diamond above.

Move the diamond across the labial surface from a mesial to distal direction, following the curvature of the gingiva from the top of the mesial interproximal papillae down to the most apical extent of the free gingival margin and back up to the tip of the distal interproximal papillae. The finish line should be right at the gingival margin in most instances.

Depending on the path of insertion, it may be necessary to remove some extra tooth substance to facilitate a path of insertion from the incisal edge toward the cervical margin. If, however, the veneer does not lap the incisal edge it can be placed from the buccal direction, and removal of all convexities will not be as critical.

2. Interproximal Extension

The margin of the porcelain laminate should generally be hidden within the embrasure area. Depending on the individual form of the tooth, it is usually desirable to extend this margin about halfway into the interproximal contact area. Extension of the laminate beyond the mesiobuccal and distobuccal line angle also ensures the wraparound effect with etched resin bonds at right angles to the labial surface for increased bond strength. This is achieved with the same LVS two-grit diamond—moving the margin into this embrasure area and just lingual to the buccal surface of the interproximal papillae so that it will not be visible from the lateral oblique view or directly from the front.

For the technician it is also useful to have extra reduction in this embrasure area so as to facilitate the addition of porcelain bulk in this region and the strengthening of the laminate around the whole periphery (i.e., interproximal areas, the incisal edge, and the cervical region). Fortunately, the interproximal areas have a thicker dimension of available enamel to allow for this slightly more extensive preparation.

Treatment of Contact Areas

The second aspect of the interproximal extension is predicated upon the type of porcelain laminate fabrication technique to be used. If the platinum foil matrix system is used, as opposed to the refractory die technique (see chapter 6), work on individual dies will be necessary. The technician will have to section the master cast by sawing from the apical end of the model toward the incisal edge but stopping short of the contact point where the saw blade would damage the teeth. If the contacts have been modified, the model can be snapped apart, separating it into individual dies. The process will require modifying the contacts prior to impression making by passing a very fine, one-sided diamond abrasive strip (Compostrip, Premier Dental Products, Norristown, Pa., 20- to 60-μm grit size) through the adjacent teeth. *The abrasive strip is used in an S configuration so that the abrasive side will reshape the contact areas rather than separate them.* Thus, a thinner contact is maintained, as measured in a buccolingual dimension. The contact area is then clearly demarcated on the model, and easy, clean snapping apart of this model into dies is facilitated. Dental floss passed through these contact areas should still just catch, so the arch integrity and stability are not disturbed.

Dentin Exposure

Dentin may be exposed during tooth preparation when dealing with a labially placed tooth that needs to be brought back into harmonious alignment with the rest of the arch. A rotated tooth poses similar problems, as does the clinical situation in which there has been gingival recession when the preparation extends apically beyond the cementoenamel junction onto exposed cementum or dentin.

If the dentinal area exposed is surrounded by enamel to provide a peripheral marginal seal, it can be managed with a dentin bonding agent. This may be a conventional dentin bonding agent, a phosphorus ester of the BIS-*GMA* molecule, or one of the newer systems such as the aluminum oxalates (Tenure, Den-Mat Corp., Santa Maria, Calif.) or glutaraldehydes.

If the dentin exposure occurs at the periphery, such as the cervical region, it is advisable to prepare a little deeper into this area so that a layer of glass ionomer can be used as a base. This glass ionomer base will bond to the dentin and seal it, as opposed to a dentin bonding agent, which may only adhere but not seal effectively. The glass ionomer can subsequently be etched concomitantly with the enamel when placing the veneer, and the composite resin luting agent will then bond to it.

Another typical example of when glass ionomer can be effectively used is cervical erosion. The eroded area already provides the depth necessary for the material. An added advantage in using the glass ionomer in these situations is the anti-caries effect offered by the continuous liberation of fluoride ions.

All dentin should be protected from the effects of the enamel etching agents (orthophosphoric acid 30% to 38%). During the enamel etching procedures use a gel form of the acid and confine it solely to the enamel. If in doubt cover the dentin with a film of dentin bonding agent (Dentin Adhesit, Vivadent, Tonawanda, N.Y.) to seal it prior to acid etching.

3. Sulcular Extension and Marginal Placement

At this stage the preparation ends right at the gingival margin. It is, however, desirable to place it *just* within the sulcus. There is no reason to *bury* it and try to hide it subgingivally, as with some crown-and-bridge procedures. The porcelain with the underlying composite resin will blend in harmoniously with the rest of the tooth without showing a cement line or metal margin. There is really no need to go any more than 0.05 to 0.1 mm into the sulcus or even to remain supragingival if a dramatic color change is not a high priority.

Sulcular extension and marginal placement are carried out with the LVS two-grit diamond described earlier. Place a narrow gingival displacement cord in the sulcus for about eight to ten

minutes to slightly displace the tissue. This system of first developing a preparation line confluent with the gingival margin and then placing a retraction cord prior to refining and extending it into the sulcus ensures (1) access for the diamond, (2) less gingival trauma, and (3) direct vision of the margin during all procedures. Because of the tissue displacement, this refined margin will appear to be supragingival until the effect of the astringent wears off. This sulcular preparation remains a considerable distance from the biologic width so there is little potential for violating it and developing untoward gingival reactions.

The margin must remain at a point where, with regard to tissue displacement, it will once again be visible for finishing of the porcelain laminate and the resin luting agent.

This region of the sulcus also has the least potential for inducing gingival reaction because the sulcular supporting enamel has not been tampered with and the subgingival coronal contour remains the same. It is a much more conservative sulcular extension than any crown-and-bridge preparation where even the all-ceramic crown invariably has an opaque cementing medium that has to be hidden below the gingival tissue.

This conservative sulcular preparation also helps ensure that the finish line does not approach the cementoenamel junction, where there may be little enamel thickness left to etch and seal the laminate to. The fine diamond at the tip of the LVS two-grit diamond cuts very slowly, thus reducing the risk of overpreparation when entering the sulcus. The diamond merely refines and defines the finish line, and in doing so it moves the finish line from being right at the gingival margin to being 0.2 mm or less into the sulcus.

Tetracycline-Stained Teeth

Tetracycline-stained teeth present a special problem that necessitates placing the finish line further subgingivally. This is done in an attempt to hide the dark discoloration that tends to show through the marginal tissue. If the enamel is penetrated through to the dentin, it is still important to at least seal the periphery of the laminate to enamel. The problem with tetracycline stain is that it is usually darkest in the cervical region where there is decreased amount of enamel to cover the stained dentin or for adequate tooth reduction. The tooth also appears darker as the enamel is removed, exposing the underlying stained dentin.

Finish Line Configuration

The actual configuration of the finish line is somewhat controversial, in that everything from a feather edge through to a rounded shoulder has been advocated.

From a purely periodontal point of view, it would be considerably better to have continuity in form from the existing enamel extending out over the new veneer; for example, there should be a continuation of the emergence profile so that there is no ledge at the junction of the veneer and the enamel to act as a depository area for microbial plaque. Thus, the finish line should involve some definitive reduction to facilitate fabrication of a veneer of sufficient thickness and strength without adding excessive contour to this sensitive region. The nature of the porcelain material and the laminate fabrication technique requires a cervical reduction of at least 0.25 mm.

A feather or knife edge finish line is the most conservative preparation but is inordinately complex because of:

1. The difficulty in fabricating porcelain to the required degree of thinness accurately—there is invariably a poor marginal fit or seal

2. The inevitable increased thickness subgingivally and resultant potential for gingival problems

3. Laboratory problems in delineating the exact end of preparation line

It would appear that the most desired form of finish line is a modified chamfer as created by the LVS two-grit diamond or one of similar shape. This modified chamfer preparation is of nominal depth (± 0.25 mm) near the cementoenamel junction where the thickness of the enamel decreases rapidly. The sulcular extension should therefore be ultra conservative in that there is an ever-decreasing thickness of available enamel as the finish line moves subgingival and approaches the cementoenamel junction.

The preparation of a chamfer in this cervical area also aids in sealing the restoration by removing the acid-resistant surface enamel and exposing subsurface enamel which is more readily etched. The modified chamfer as developed by the two-grit diamond seems to be the preparation of choice.

Benefits of the Modified Chamfer Finish Line

- An increased bulk of porcelain at the margin and hence increased strength without overcontour

- Correct enamel preparation exposing correctly aligned enamel rods for increased bond strength at the cervical margin

- A well-defined finish line for the laboratory yet without too great a potential for porcelain sintering shrinkage—increased accuracy of fit

- Greater ease for the dentist to obtain a correct gingival finish line after insertion

- A definitive stop to aid in seating the laminate in the correct position on the tooth

- An accurately fitting restoration with sound marginal seal due to the use of the fine-grit diamond at the tip of the two-grit bur

4. Incisal or Occlusal Reduction

The fabrication of a porcelain veneer lapping the incisal edge makes placement of the restoration that much easier by virtue of having a definitive stop during seating. The incisal edge gives the clinician a specific relationship from which to evaluate whether the restoration is correctly positioned. This incisal overlap can even be fabricated purely as a positioning device and then later removed once the veneer is bonded in place. This latter type of incisal extension requires no real preparation because the overlap will be ground away following luting and placement of the laminate.

There are times, however, when added length may be desirable, and in these situations it is necessary to actually prepare the incisal aspect of the tooth. The preparation should be a definitive flattening of the incisal edge to create increased enamel width and potential bonding surface for the laminate. The sharp line angles created on the buccal and lingual surfaces must be rounded, however, which will again increase the surface area of enamel and prevent the propagation of microcracks in the porcelain.

The reduction should be at least 1 mm if it is desired to restore the original length. Simple reshaping of the edge as described above without vertical reduction will suffice if the teeth are to be lengthened.

If the incisal edge is not to be included it is still useful to increase the amount of horizontal tooth reduction at the periphery of the preparation, the interproximal areas, and the incisal edge. This will give the technician extra space to stack porcelain and so develop a thicker periphery for strength. Safer handling at a later stage by the clinician is also facilitated. The incisal edge is thus hollowed out slightly for a dimension of 0.2 mm creating this space.

In general, never end the incisal edge where excursive movements of the mandible will cause shearing stresses across the junction of porcelain laminate and tooth. This potentiates fracture of the porcelain, debonding, and ongoing exposure of the composite resin in this crucial area.

5. Lingual Reduction

Any reduction of the incisal edge may necessitate some lingual enamel modification so that there is no butt joint at this incisal/lingual junction but rather a rounded chamfer. This modification will help to prevent the porcelain from shearing away from the incisal edge during function. It also ensures *(1)* increased thickness of porcelain in this critical lingual area that is being used for incising and guidance, *(2)* enamel bonds at right angles to those on the incisal edge, and *(3)* increased strength.

Excessive buccal convexity of a tooth may make it difficult to overlap the incisal edge and still maintain an incisal path of insertion. An excessive amount of labial tooth structure may have to be removed to facilitate a path of insertion, thereby exposing large amounts of dentin. In these situations the veneer should be designed to rotate about a more rounded incisal preparation in seating it. It is not advisable to compromise and have a butt porcelain joint on the lingual incisal line angle to facilitate a buccal path of insertion. The shearing force will peel this margin open in protrusive movements of the mandible.

Before impressions are made, reevaluate the enamel reduction for the following:

- Even and adequate overall reduction
- Definitive smooth finish line—modified chamfer if desired
- A simple path of insertion with no undercuts
- Rounded line angles
- Modification of the contact areas

The final decision on whether or not to perform enamel reduction remains a clinical chairside decision. It must be based on the following criteria:

1. The relative position of the teeth in the arch. Malpositioned and rotated teeth may need reduction to bring them within the confines of the arch.

2. The color of the teeth to be veneered. Darkly stained teeth often require more reduction for opaquing purposes.

3. The propensity for overcontouring to induce gingival problems due to microbial plaque accumulation. If the laminate ends supragingivally it may be considerably easier to maintain this interface plaque free.

4. Partial coverage veneers as in closure of diastemata may require little or no preparation.

5. The patient's age, relative size of tooth pulps, and psychological approach to tooth reduction.

The dentist should also evaluate the patient and his or her individual expectations. If a patient is apprehensive and unsure then it is wise to perform no reduction, leaving the clinician the option, if necessary, of grinding away the porcelain veneer and repolishing the enamel, thereby returning the patient to a semblance of his or her original state, although this is a most difficult task.

An Atlas of Enamel Reduction

Labial Reduction
(Figs. 4-8 to 4-14)

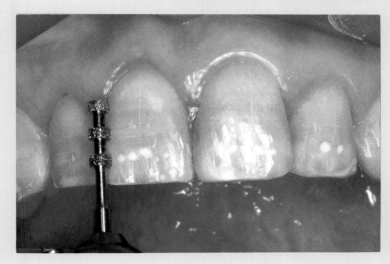

Fig. 4-8 Place the two-grit diamond on the distal aspect of the maxillary left central incisor and draw it across toward the opposite interproximal area.

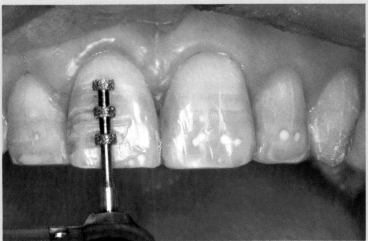

Fig. 4-9 The diamond will develop striations to the required depth on the labial face of the tooth.

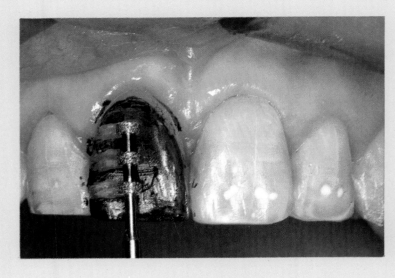

Fig. 4-10 To highlight the effect in Fig. 4-8, the rest of the tooth has been colored green. Draw the bur across the tooth the rest of the way toward the opposite interproximal area.

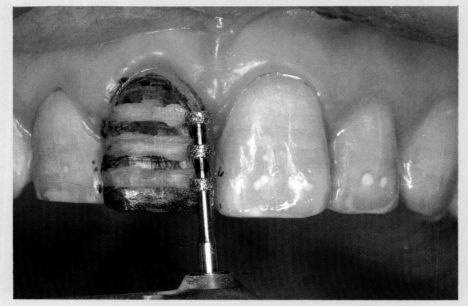

Fig. 4-11 The bur has been drawn across the complete labial surface of the tooth and the depth-cut striations are evident as white lines against the green background.

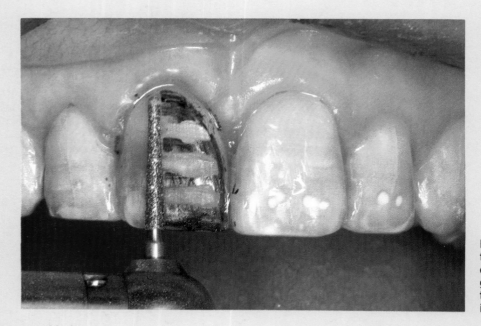

Fig. 4-12 Utilize the two-grit diamond to reduce the remaining green-colored enamel to the depth of the horizontal striations.

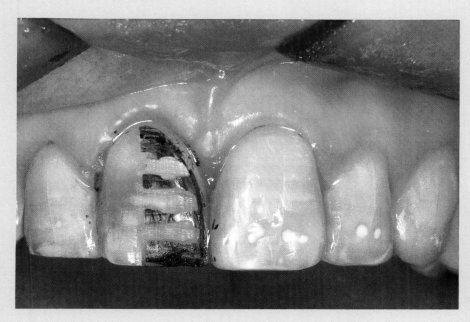

Fig. 4-13 The distal aspect of the tooth has been reduced to the depth of the depth-cut striations. The mesial half of the tooth still has the grooves and remaining enamel present.

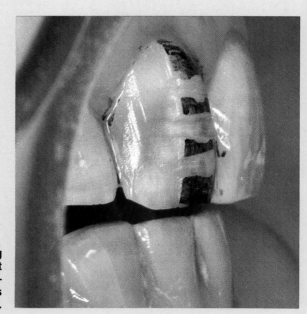

Fig. 4-14 Lateral oblique view showing depth-cut striations on the distal aspect of the tooth with remaining green-colored enamel and depth-cut striations interspersed.

Interproximal Extension
(Figs. 4-15 to 4-17)

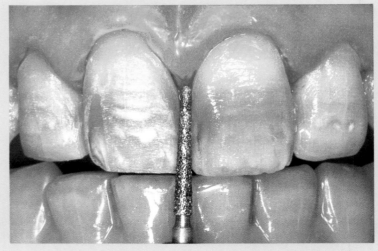

Fig. 4-15 Utilize the two-grit diamond to enhance the reduction in the interproximal areas and increase the potential thickness of porcelain.

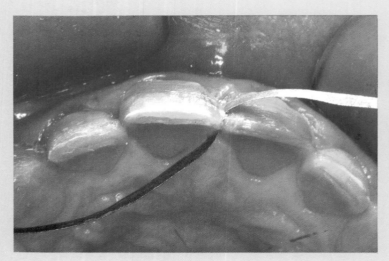

Fig. 4-16 Utilize the abrasive strip to accentuate the demarcation of the contact areas by reducing the lingual aspect of the interproximal contact point. This will maintain the contact points but will make them somewhat more V-shaped and well demarcated.

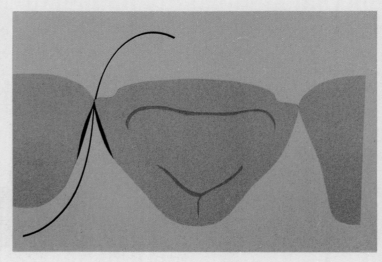

Fig. 4-17 Diagram indicating correct use of abrasive strip and reshaped lingual interproximal enamel; however, contact point is maintained.

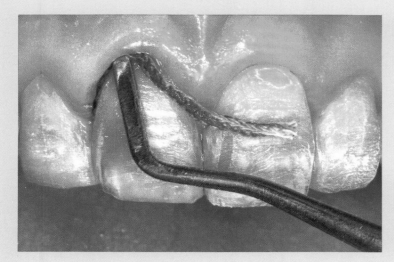

Sulcular Marginal Placement
(Figs. 4-18 to 4-20)

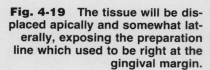

Fig. 4-18 The teeth have been prepared on the labial aspect so that the finish line is exactly at the gingival margin. Place a thin, braided, gingival retraction cord lightly into the sulcus.

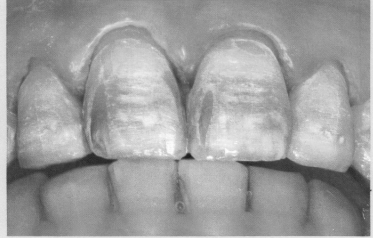

Fig. 4-19 The tissue will be displaced apically and somewhat laterally, exposing the preparation line which used to be right at the gingival margin.

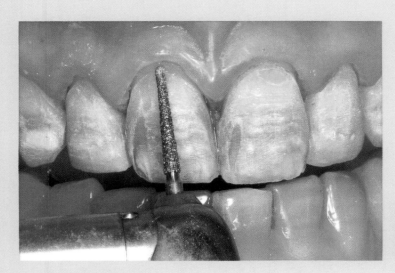

Fig. 4-20 Use the tip of the two-grit diamond to *refine and define this finish line without moving it apically,* if possible. Ensure that it is a smooth harmonious finish line.

Incisal/Lingual Reduction
(Figs. 4-21 to 4-23)

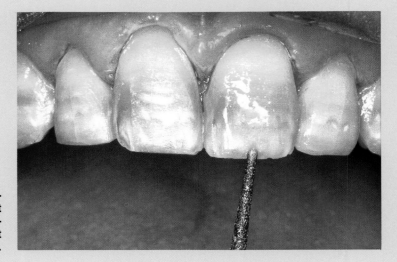

Fig. 4-21 Use the two-grit diamond to enhance the reduction at the incisal edge to facilitate increased porcelain thickness at the peripheral area.

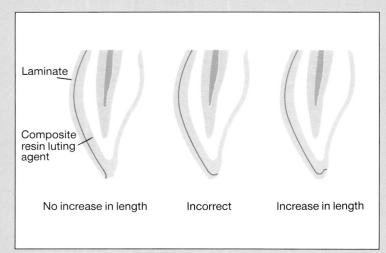

Laminate

Composite
resin luting
agent

No increase in length   Incorrect   Increase in length

Fig. 4-22 *(left)* Incisal design when no increase in tooth length is desired. *(middle)* Incorrect design of incisal preparation if increase in tooth length is desired. Incorrect finish line; butt joint susceptible to opening during protrusive movement of mandible. *(right)* Correct form for incisal preparation when increase in tooth length is desired. Lingual chamfer results in increased strength due to being at a right angle and parallel to protrusive motion of mandible.

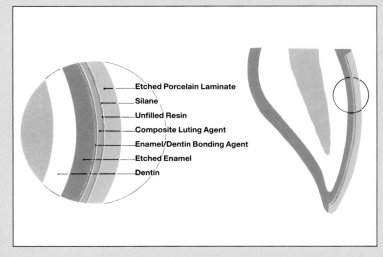

Etched Porcelain Laminate
Silane
Unfilled Resin
Composite Luting Agent
Enamel/Dentin Bonding Agent
Etched Enamel
Dentin

Fig. 4-23 Cross-section diagram depicting tooth preparation.

Bibliography

Albers, H.F. Tooth Colored Restoratives. 7th ed. Cotati, Calif.: Alto Books, 1985.

Feinman, R.A. A combination therapy. CDA Journal April, 1987, pp. 10–13.

Friedman, M. Personal communication, 1985.

Ibsen, R. The New Cosmetic Dentistry Syllabus. Santa Maria, Calif.: Den-Mat Corp., 1987.

Jordan, R.E. Esthetic Composite Bonding. Toronto, Philadelphia: B.C. Decker, 1986.

Nixon, R.L. The Chairside Manual for Porcelain Bonding. Wilmington, Del.: B.A. Videographics, 1987.

Impressions and Temporization

5

The fabrication of porcelain laminate veneers necessitates some form of a master cast. This cast must be an accurate reproduction of what exists in the mouth, and the impression material should be selected from among those that are used for any crown-and-bridge technique. Commonly used materials include polysulfide, polyether, and vinyl polysiloxane elastomeric, and hydrocolloid impression materials. Although most any crown-and-bridge material can be used, hydrocolloid tends to tear in the unprepared undercut areas below or between the contact areas. These undercut areas are normally removed in conventional crown preparations; therefore, an elastomeric material with greater tensile strength is more desirable. The detail obtained by an alginate impression is probably not of sufficient quality to ensure a precise fit of the laminate.

Prior to deciding upon the type of impression material to be used, the laboratory laminate fabrication technique should be determined. The **platinum foil technique** uses individual removable dies on a master cast made up of conventional die stone. The die stone can easily be poured into any of the above mentioned impression materials, rendering an accurate reproduction of the tooth preparation. It should be noted, though, that for this system the master cast will have to be separated into individual dies. Good delineation of each tooth is ensured if the contact points in the mouth are modified by shaping with an ultra-fine diamond strip (Compostrip, Premier Dental Products, Norristown, Pa.) so that dental floss still slightly catches (see chapter 3).

In the **refractory technique,** the die material employed is a phosphate-bonded refractory investment. This cannot be used with a hydrocolloid impression because it will distort during the exothermic setting process of the investment. Instead, this technique necessitates that one of the elastomeric impression materials such as a vinyl polysiloxane be utilized.

In refractory-technique cases it may be prudent to block out lingual interproximal undercut areas with orthodontic wax. *Never do this if the foil technique is being used because the technician will not be able to section the model.* In the refractory-technique case, it may even be adequate to remove the lingual flange of the tray and only take a buccoincisal impression.

These two techniques are discussed in detail in chapter 6.

In most situations the impression will be sent to the laboratory so that the technicians can pour up the model themselves. Hydrocolloids necessitate being poured immediately; also, because of their nature, the laboratory technicians cannot make more than one pour in each impression. The elastomeric material is more advantageous, because it maintains its dimensional stability during travel and can be poured two times or more.

The impression material either can be utilized in a conventional type of tray or, to save time, a combined maxillary/mandibular bite tray system may be used.

Impression Technique

Tissue Management

The preparation finish line is right at the gingival margin, delineating the periphery of the laminate. Displace the tissue so that the final finish line can be seen in the sulcus (Fig. 5-1). Tissue displacement is readily accomplished with fine cotton cord impregnated with an astringent agent such as aluminum sulfate (Hemodent, Premier Dental Products, Norristown, Pa.). This procedure will displace tissue laterally and provide access to the sulcus, thereby allowing the operator to visualize the refinement of the final finish line just within the sulcus.

Gently tuck the retraction cord into the sulcus. Forces in excess of 5 g should not be employed so as not to disrupt the integrity of the junctional epithelium. The cord should extend from the interproximal mesial surface around the labial sur-

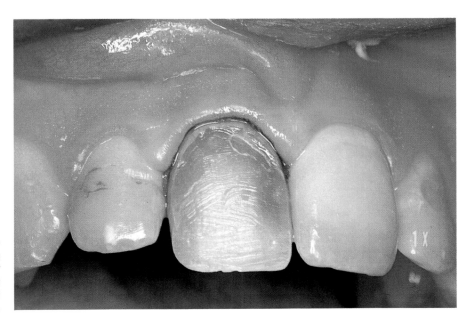

Fig. 5-1 Prior to making the impression, the tooth is prepared for the laminate. Tissue displacement cord is in place.

face and onto the distal interproximal surface. The cord needs to remain in place for some five minutes before being removed—*wet*—to avoid tearing the friable junctional epithelium and precipitating bleeding.

Impression

The impression material used should be of two viscosities: light and heavy. The tray material should be of the heavy type. The light material should either be syringed into the sulcus or, in the case of hydrocolloid, simply be placed over the preparation. This will facilitate the heavy body moving the light body up into the sulcus and embrasures, to pick up the periphery of the preparation. As with any crown-and-bridge medium and more specifically for laminates, the impression material should have high tensile strength as well as accuracy. Insert the tray from an oblique buccal direction to make certain all labial and gingival relationships are properly recorded.

Temporization

Temporization for laminates is usually unnecessary because, in most situations, only half of the enamel surface is removed and the dentinal tubules are not exposed; therefore there should be little or no sensitivity and only minimal esthetic compromise. Also, temporary veneers for the most part are undesirable because they may by their very nature cause gingival inflammation.

However, in certain situations, temporization may become necessary when teeth have been more extensively reduced to facilitate aligning of the laminates along a preexisting arch. In these situations there may be areas of exposed dentin that require temporary veneers because of sensitivity. There may also be open contacts that potentiate movement of the teeth in the interim between preparation and final insertion of the laminates. Mandibular teeth with incisal reduction should also be prevented from erupting by some form of temporary veneer. Those situations where the reduced teeth are just too unesthetic for the patient to function adequately also require temporization.

There are four basic techniques for developing the temporary veneers:

Direct Composite Resin Veneer

This system involves the placement of a composite resin restorative material directly on the *unetched* surface of the prepared teeth.

Shape the composite resin while soft with a composite resin placement instrument (GCI no. 3, GC International Corp., Scottsdale, Ariz.) and then cure it with the respective light. It can then be trimmed with a high-speed handpiece and composite resin finishing burs (E.T. Burs, Bras-

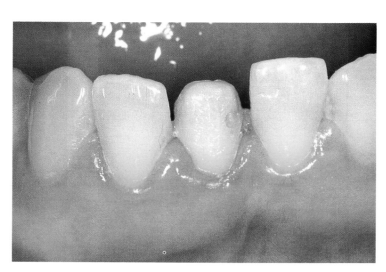

Fig. 5-2 The mandibular left central incisor is prepared for the porcelain laminate.

seler, Savannah, Ga.) into the correct form as dictated by the adjacent teeth and occlusion (Figs. 5-2 and 5-3).

In general there is no need to etch the prepared tooth or to use any form of bonding agent in order to maintain the temporary composite resin laminate in place. However, in certain situations it may be necessary to spot etch a small area in the *center* of the labial surface and use a bonding agent to improve retention. ***It is essential to ensure that the periphery of the preparation is not involved or compromised by etching.*** The temporary veneer is removed by prying it away from the tooth or by grinding it away with a high-speed handpiece and diamond stone until fresh enamel is reached. The extra amount of enamel removed is inconsequential and readily compensated for by the composite resin luting agent. The unetched peripheral composite resin will come off, leaving an uncompromised marginal area.

The direct composite resin system will work nicely for one or two individual units, but it may be too time-consuming when doing four or more laminates.

Direct Composite Resin Veneer Utilizing Vacuform Matrix

In this technique, the vacuform matrix is made up on a preoperative plaster cast of the patient's mouth (Figs. 5-4 and 5-5). This cast may be altered and reshaped into a more esthetic form in the laboratory prior to forming the plastic matrix.

Separate the clear vacuform matrix from the cast and trim it. Scallop the area around the gingival margins and cut it **short** of the soft tissue line and well into the interproximal areas (Fig. 5-6).

Fill the labial aspect of the vacuform with a light-cured composite resin and manipulate the whole complex gently into place on the patient's prepared teeth (Fig. 5-7). The area that has been cut away from the gingival margin allows for manipulation of the soft uncured resin into correct form so that it does not impinge upon the soft tissues and interproximal areas. Then set the composite with the appropriate light-curing unit, and peel the vacuform away from the teeth, leaving the composite resin in place. Trim and shape it to act as the interim temporary veneer using finishing burs and polishing disks (Fig. 5-8).

It is essential to ensure that the composite resin does not impinge upon the tissue in any way, otherwise untoward gingival reactions may occur. Any inflammation of the soft tissues compromises final seating of the laminates due to crevicular fluid seepage and/or hemorrhage when the tissues are even gently manipulated.

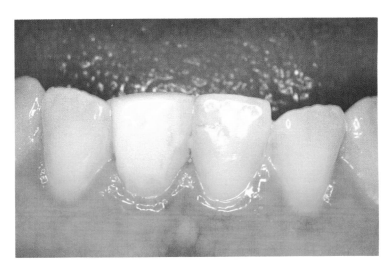

Fig. 5-3 Direct composite resin temporary veneer after two weeks.

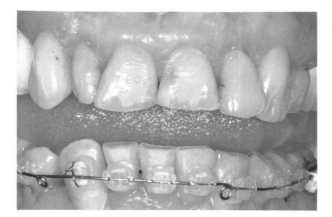

Fig. 5-4 Preoperative view of the teeth to be laminated.

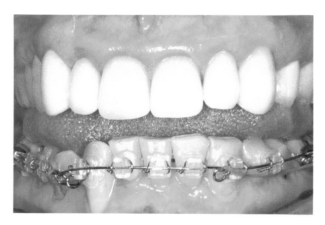

Fig. 5-5 Vacuform matrix is made to simulate desired form of final case.

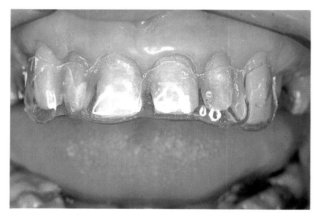

Fig. 5-6 The vacuform matrix is in position on the prepared teeth. Note that it is scalloped short of all soft tissue.

Direct Acrylic Veneer

In this technique, instead of utilizing composite resin, methyl methacrylate self-curing acrylic resin is mixed into a soupy state, flowed into the buccal aspects of the vacuform, and allowed to reach the "doughy" stage of curing.

Once in this doughy stage, manipulate the vacuform into position over the prepared teeth that have been lubricated to facilitate easy removal. Then manipulate these acrylic resin veneers in the vacuform on and off gently, allowing them to cure but not to engage in any undercuts on the prepared teeth. Remove them from the teeth and take them to the laboratory where they can be trimmed and polished, using the utmost caution not to fracture them. Either cement them into place with a laminate composite resin luting system, taking care to remove the extruded excess before light curing, or leave them as a removable temporary.

Indirect Composite Resin/Acrylic Resin Veneer

These temporary veneers are fabricated in the laboratory on a cast of the prepared teeth (Figs. 5-9 and 5-10). If an in-house laboratory exists these can be rapidly prepared on a cast of the preparations.

Gently manipulate the matrix and material into position on the cast of the prepared teeth and cure. Trim the matrix and polish it on this cast before separating (Fig. 5-11). Lute in place with any composite resin system (Fig. 5-12).

In none of the above techniques does any acid etching need to be done; hence, the temporary veneers should peel away readily at the second visit without affecting the ability to subsequently acid etch the enamel. If the temporary veneers need added adhesion, spot etch a small area in the center of the labial surface, using a gel etch for 15 seconds. An unfilled resin can then be used to tack the veneer in place. However, in most situations, this is unnecessary.

Fig. 5-7 The vacuform matrix, in position on the prepared teeth, is filled with composite resin.

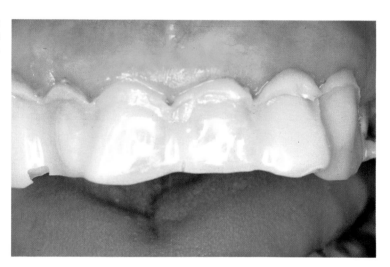

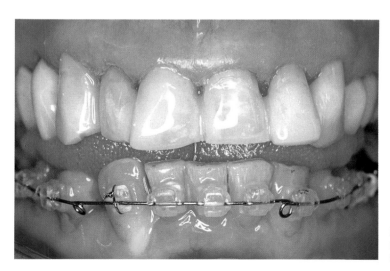

Fig. 5-8 Completed temporary resin veneers mimic the preoperative form.

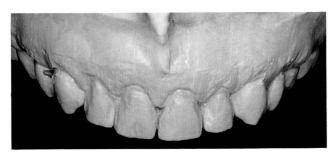

Fig. 5-9 Plaster cast of preparations for veneers.

Fig. 5-10 Acrylic temporary veneers on the plaster cast.

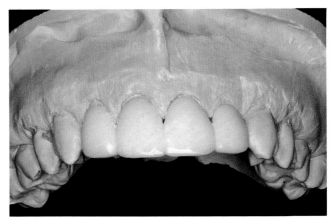

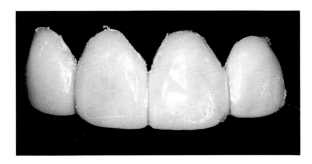

Fig. 5-11 The acrylic veneer is polished and removed from cast.

Fig. 5-12 Indirect acrylic resin veneers are luted in position with composite resin.

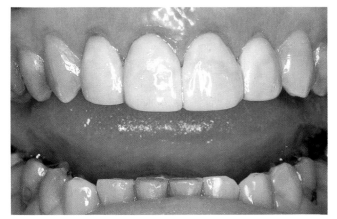

Shade Selection

In general, it is advisable to select a shade that is slightly lighter than that desired by the patient. Subtle shade modification is possible using the various composite resin systems. It is somewhat easier to darken any given shade than to lighten it. So in general, select a shade that is higher in value and lower in chroma. Shade selection for laminates varies somewhat from that of conventional crown-and-bridge techniques, where any chosen shade guide tab can be matched by the ceramist. In processing porcelain laminates, the ceramist may well be able to deliver a shade A2 veneer (Vita-Lumin, Vita Zahnfabrik, Bad Sackingen, West Germany), but once it is luted in place the final color can be very different.

The final color of the restoration will be the combined result of several factors and not only the porcelain shade selected:

- The original tooth color
- The shade selected for porcelain and amount of opacifier added
- The color and opacity of the composite resin luting agent
- The use of resin shade modifiers and characterizers behind the veneers

Laboratory Procedures

6

Thomas Greggs

Communication

In visualizing the many variables that will have an impact on the final appearance and esthetic value of the finished porcelain veneer, the ceramist will need to make use of all relevant information. Laboratory prescription forms, if used correctly, are an excellent communication vehicle between dentist and laboratory technician. They can provide all pertinent information and anecdotal comments. These accurate descriptions should supplement and accompany (1) a good impression, (2) bite registration, (3) cast of opposing arch, and (4) shade selection. Photographs are also an excellent aid to the technician. They can convey important information regarding the preexisting shade of the teeth, the lip line, the location and color of any discoloration or stain, and the relative position of the teeth, gingivae, and lips. Finally, it may also be helpful to provide a diagnostic wax-up or a computer-generated diagnostic printout.

Accurate color evaluation of the tooth or teeth to be veneered and the shade relationship to adjacent teeth is crucial to maximizing esthetics of the finished veneer. Shade selection should be made with a tendency to select a lighter color. This is because it is easier to darken, rather than lighten, overall color with use of the underlying composite resin. Severely discolored teeth can be more predictably masked by using opacifiers within the porcelain itself. The clinician is then less dependent upon the thin layer of luting resin for the modification of color.

A key advantage of porcelain veneers is that they are fabricated indirectly in a laboratory. They utilize the ceramist's expertise in creating a realistic restoration yet still allow the dentist the opportunity to individualize and characterize the veneer through chairside shade techniques and cosmetic contouring.

Two diverse laboratory techniques for fabrication of porcelain veneers have gained wide acceptance:

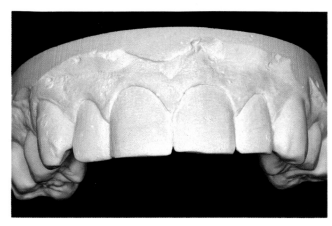

Fig. 6-1 A master cast of hard die stone is shown, trimmed and ready for use.

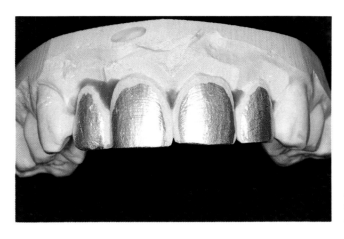

Fig. 6-2 Master cast with die spacer correctly applied. Block-out wax has been placed to fill in any undercuts.

1. The refractory investment technique

2. The platinum foil technique

Both methods, if handled judiciously, will produce clinically acceptable, esthetic veneers. The two methods presented are patented techniques (U.S. Pat. No. 3,986,261; U.S. Pat. No. 4,473,353; U.S. Pat. No. 4,579,530).

The Refractory Investment Technique

1. Fabrication of a Master Cast

A hard die stone, of crown-and-bridge standards, should be chosen for pouring the master cast. Before the stone model is poured, treat the impression with a liquid to reduce surface tension between the impression and the die stone. This will decrease the occurrence of air bubbles while the master cast is poured. Carefully pour the die stone into the impression and allow it to bench set for 30 minutes. When the stone is completely set, release the stone master cast from the impression and allow it to dry and harden further (Fig. 6-1).

2. Application of Die Spacer

Before beginning the fabrication of the refractory model, but only if deemed necessary, carefully apply a thin layer of die spacer to the labial surfaces of the prepared teeth on the master cast. This will allow space for the film thickness of the luting resin when the veneer is bonded to the tooth. The die spacer should be kept clear of the margins (Fig. 6-2). Caution should be used when choosing to use a die spacer, since adequate space (15 to 20 μm) for the composite resin material will be developed during the subsequent steps of veneer fabrication (i.e., application of ceramic sealant, air abrasion, and etching the inner surface of veneer). A die spacer should therefore be considered only if additional space (0.1 mm) for underlying composite resin is needed, as in the case of a badly discolored tooth, where the dentist desires to do his or her own opaquing at the time of insertion. Too great a thickness of composite resin may weaken the final restoration. This is because it is not as rigid a material as porcelain. It is generally more desirable to have as thin a film of composite resin as possible via a well-fitting laminate.

3. Fabrication of Refractory Model

A refractory investment material should be chosen with a coefficient of thermal expansion similar to that of the ceramic being used for the porcelain veneer. If the difference in coefficients of thermal expansion is too great between the refractory die material and the ceramic, there is a risk of disproportionate expansion during processing of the porcelain. Improper fit of the veneer to the tooth, or even fracture of the restorations, will result.

Select a preformed plastic disposable tray to fit on the master cast over the teeth to be veneered. Only a labial-incisal impression will be taken of this area. Cut away the lingual flange on the impression tray and the tray material distal to the last tooth being veneered (Fig. 6-3).

Survey the master cast for undercut areas. These should be blocked out at this time to allow for subsequent placement and fitting of the finished veneer. Working with a master cast that is completely dry, use an oil base block-out wax to fill in any undercuts in embrasure areas or on the labial surface. Before the refractory impression is taken, thinly coat the master cast with a silicone-based lubricant. This will facilitate easy removal of the tray impression material. Mix an elastomeric impression material and place it into the custom-cut plastic tray, then take an impression of the labial-incisal areas to be veneered (Fig. 6-4). (Follow respective manufacturers' recommended directions for use of the impression material.)

When the labial impression has set on the master cast, submerge both in water, where they can be more easily separated. Check the impression for any relevant air bubbles or discrepancies and adjust. Pour it into the labial impression, and allow it to bench set. The manufacturer's directions for correct powder:liquid ratio and setting time should be precisely followed.

Once the refractory model is completely dry, release the model from the impression while submerged in water which, again, allows for easier separation (Fig. 6-5). A second refractory model may be poured, following the same procedure used with the first refractory model.

The refractory models should be *dry trimmed*. This method avoids surface discrepancies that can develop due to the slurry created with wet trimming.

4. Preparation of Refractory Model

The porcelain veneers may be built on either a solid refractory model or on individual refractory dies taken from two refractory models. If using individual refractory dies, specifically section two refractory models to develop single dies from every alternate tooth of the two models. In this way, each refractory individual die to be veneered will be built to full contour from one of the two models.

Whether using a solid refractory model or separate refractory dies, undercut the die stem apical to the cervical margin, trim away the gingival area, and eliminate the interdental papillae. The finish line will then be defined distinctly. Care must be taken not to abrade the contact areas. The solid refractory cast or individual dies are reduced below the gingival margin 13 to 19 mm to allow for easier handling. The lingual base area is trimmed no more than 13 mm from the labial surface to the firing tray, as measured when the refractory model is placed with the lingual base on the firing tray.

Minimizing the bulk of the refractory investment allows for easier handling. It also leaves less investment material to be de-gassed and facilitates a more uniform firing of the investment material and ceramic.

5. De-Gassing the Refractory Investment

To avoid contamination of the ceramic, ammon-

Fig. 6-3 Cut a preformed plastic disposable tray to fit over the master cast to include the area being veneered and the teeth adjacent to it.

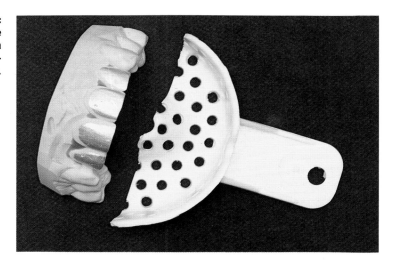

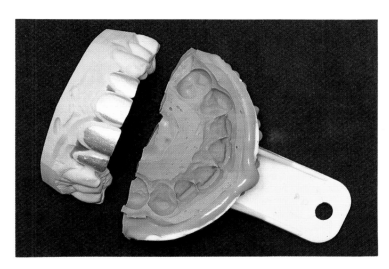

Fig. 6-4 Make an impression of the master cast using an elastomeric impression material. The impression must accurately reproduce the labial-incisal areas to be veneered.

Fig. 6-5 A refractory model is made from the labial impression of the master cast. Since the veneers will be built upon refractory material it must be of a similar coefficient of thermal expansion as the ceramic selected to fabricate the veneers.

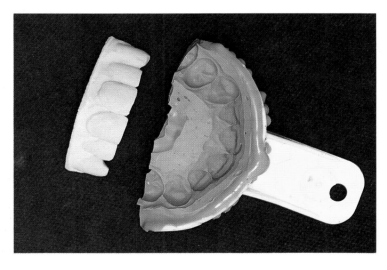

iated gasses inherent in the refractory material must be removed. Manufacturers' de-gassing procedures should be followed specifically for the chosen investment material. The basic procedure is as follows:

1. Introduce the refractory model to the pre-heated furnace at low temperatures ranging from 1,000°F (540°C) to 1,200°F (650°C) and heat-soak it for 15 to 30 minutes.

2. Then place the model under vacuum and set the temperature between 1,900°F (1,040°C) to 1,950°F (1,066°C) with a heat rate increase of 75°F (25°C) per minute.

3. Hold the temperature at 1,900°F (1,040°C)to 1,950°F (1,066°C) for two to six minutes.

4. Release the vacuum with a slow decline in temperature to approximately 1,000°F (540°C).

5. Remove the refractory model (or dies) from the furnace and bench cool them.

It is advisable that an auxiliary furnace be strictly utilized for the de-gas/heat–soak procedure, because long-term exposure to ammo-niated gasses may cause problems in a furnace used for other purposes too. (Be sure to closely follow individual manufacturer's instructions.)

6. Sealant Application

So that the refractory investment will not absorb moisture from the porcelain mix, a specific refractory sealant may be placed over all porcelain bearing surfaces and marginal areas. Any sealant may be chosen from a variety available on the market, or a slurried mix of the veneering porcelain can be applied to the porcelain-bearing surfaces.

Soak the refractory dies in distilled water for four to five minutes. Prepare the sealant, or wet slurry of porcelain, and paint it over the moist (but not wet) porcelain-bearing surfaces of the die. The sealant must be applied beyond the labial margins to achieve a good peripheral seal. Then fire the painted refractory model, or dies, according to the firing cycle of the porcelain being used. When the refractory model is removed from the furnace it should have a sheen to the surface. If not, repeat the procedure of sealing (Fig. 6-6).

The porcelain is built up to full contour and the veneers are finished and contoured prior to stain

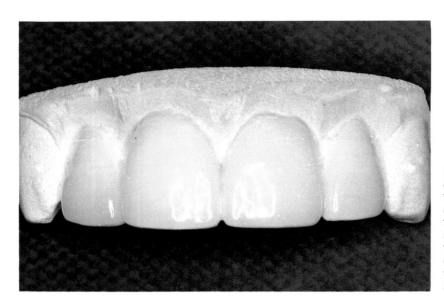

Fig. 6-6 Following the application of a die sealer, the porcelain is applied and fired. Here, a case of four anterior teeth is shown, built on a solid refractory model. Facial anatomy will be redefined before staining and glazing are completed.

application and glazing (see following individual sections on "porcelain buildup," "finishing and contouring," and "glazing").

7. Removal of Veneers from Refractory Material

After the veneers are glazed and bench cooled, carefully trim the refractory investment material with an appropriate bur until only a minimal amount of refractory material remains around the veneers (Fig. 6-7). Air abrade the refractory cast with 20 to 50 μm particles of aluminum oxide at 60 psi to remove the refractory material from the interface of the veneer (Fig. 6-8).

Carefully remove and clean the veneers in an ultrasonic detergent bath for three minutes. Use a rubber wheel to lightly remove all porcelain flash and overextensions from the edges before returning the veneers to the master cast for adjustment (Figs. 6-9 and 6-10) (see following sections on "adjustment and placement on master model" and "etching").

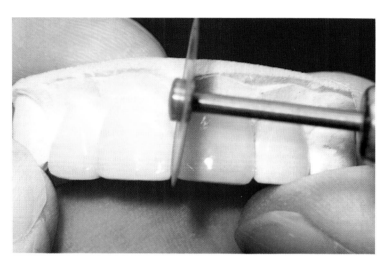

Fig. 6-7 Use an ultrathin diamond disk to separate the veneers while they are on the refractory model.

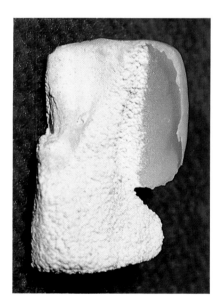

Fig. 6-8 Carefully trim away the refractory material at the gingival margin with a double-sided cutting disk. A bur will remove the bulk of refractory material from the interface of the veneer. Any remaining refractory material is removed by air abrading with 50 μm particles of aluminum oxide at 60 psi, as shown after partial air abrasion.

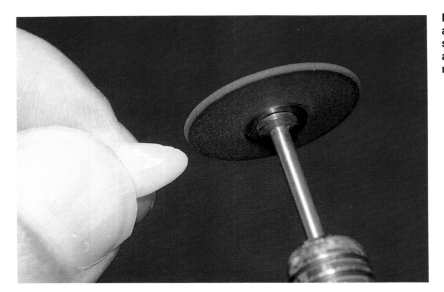

Fig. 6-9 Lightly remove any flash and overextensions using a rubber wheel around the edges of the veneer.

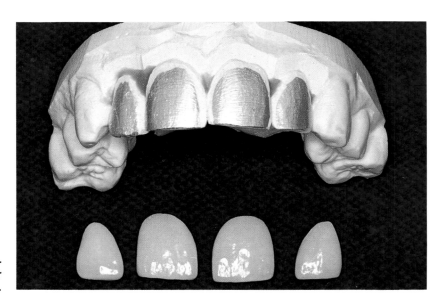

Fig. 6-10 Return the veneers to the master cast for final adjustments.

Platinum Foil Technique

1. Choosing a Foil

Platinum foil commonly used for veneering is 0.001 to 0.00085 in. in thickness, and is usually sold in widths of $1\frac{1}{6}$ to $1\frac{3}{8}$ in. However, the handling characteristics of different manufacturer's platinum foil may vary. Some types of foil at the same thickness are stiffer and less pliable than others. For this reason, it is recommended that a foil designed specifically for fabrication of porcelain veneers be used to ensure reliable handling characteristics and predictable results (P.V.S. Laboratory Kit, Cercom International, Wheaton, Ill.). The platinum foil not only acts as a surface substrate for veneer buildup but also serves to radiate heat during firing, bringing the entire porcelain to a uniform maturity.

When foil is peeled away from the interface of the finished veneer, the interface will have a smooth, glaze-like surface before it is etched and air abraded. Therefore, it is advantageous to use a porcelain with maximum capacity for etching.

2. Model and Die Preparation

Starting with a good quality elastomeric impression, use a hard dental die stone to pour a working model. Build up a base of at least 10 mm from the gingival margin and trim it when the model is set. Using a reliable pin system, pin all teeth to be veneered, including the adjacent teeth. To further stabilize the dies and ensure accuracy, a double pinning technique is recommended (Fig. 6-11). Pour the base (following the manufacturer's instructions), allow it to harden, and then trim it.

Section and cut individual dies from the master cast. This is done by sectioning the cast from the base toward the incisal edge but stopping short of the contact points (Figs. 6-12 and 6-13). The saw blades available are too thick to cut through incisally without destroying the contact of the dies. Once the contact area is reached, snap apart the cast (Fig. 6-14). (This is facilitated by the clinician modifying the contact points, as described in chapter 3.) Use a no. 8 round bur to undercut the die at the gingival and proximal margins. Re-move excess stone from the base of the dies to create a smooth, rounded shape, providing easy access to the working surface of the die (Fig. 6-15). Cover all undercuts and enamel flaws with a block-out wax to facilitate easy removal of the foil (Fig. 6-16).

3. Foil Matrix

With a triangular template specifically designed for veneering, cut the foil into the designated shape (Fig. 6-17). Place it over the labial surface of the die with the apex pointing downward, thus forming a tab portion which extends below the gingival margin (Fig. 6-18). Systematically wrap the foil over the incisal edge and into the undercuts of the gingival/proximal margins (Figs. 6-19 and 6-20). Methodically using an orangewood stick, adapt and burnish the foil into an intimately fitting form (Fig. 6-21). The excess foil on the proximal surfaces beyond the margins must be trimmed away using a scalpel. The prepared platinum foil can be seen in Fig. 6-22.

An alternative process involves "swaging" the platinum foil. In this procedure, the foil is adapted to the die, lightly burnished, wrapped with a protective sheet of plastic, and positioned in a swaging apparatus. Force is exerted onto the apparatus to mold the foil to the die as it is forced into the swaging clay. The die is dislodged from the swaging apparatus and the plastic wrap removed, leaving a foil very closely adapted to the die.

When using either method of foil adaptation, the excess foil at the proximal margins must be trimmed away. To remove the foil matrix from the die, carefully lift the tab extension from the gingival surface toward the incisal surface in a hinge-like fashion (Fig. 6-23). Hold this foil matrix over a Bunsen burner flame until it glows bright orange, to decontaminate and anneal it (Fig. 6-24). The decontaminated foil is then readapted to the die and secured with several peripherally placed drops of sticky wax (Fig. 6-25). Mix and apply the preselected porcelain shades to the platinum foil following the suggested buildup technique (see following section on "porcelain application"). Fire the porcelain according to manufacturer's instructions. Complete finishing and glazing (Figs. 6-26 to 6-35) (see following sections on "finishing and contouring" and "glazing").

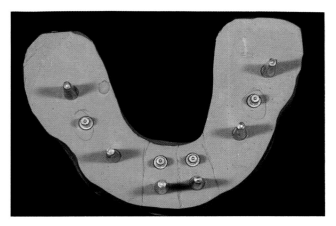

Figs. 6-11 to 6-36 courtesy of Pinhas Adar.

Fig. 6-11 Master cast showing double pinning system.

Fig. 6-12 The cavosurface margin is demarcated in red pencil. This delineates all the area to be covered by the laminate.

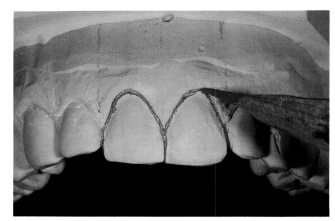

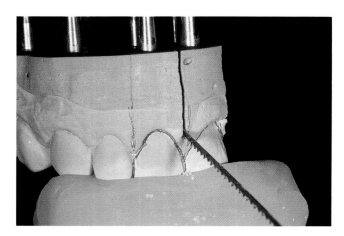

Fig. 6-13 Saw down through the model from the apical end toward the contact point, stopping before the blade impinges upon the teeth on either side.

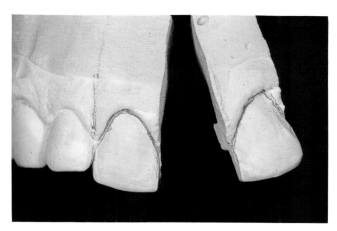

Fig. 6-14 The model can now be snapped apart by virtue of the decrease in buccolingual contact area width. This modification is developed by the clinician during the tooth preparation phase utilizing ultrathin metal strips (see Figs. 4-16 and 4-17).

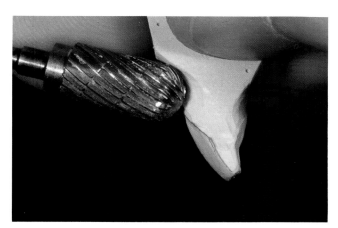

Fig. 6-15 Remove the excess die material to demarcate the cavosurface margin.

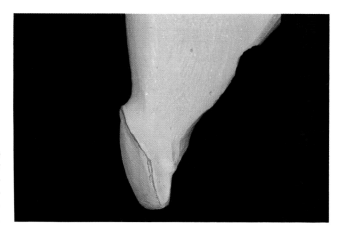

Fig. 6-16 Lateral view of the die showing how the periphery of the preparation is demarcated and the diestem is undercut to facilitate easy removal of the foil.

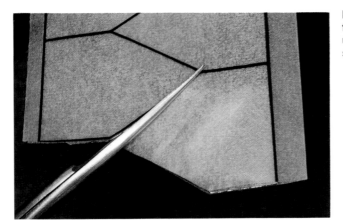

Fig. 6-17 Cut the platinum foil into the necessary shape utilizing the specifically designed template.

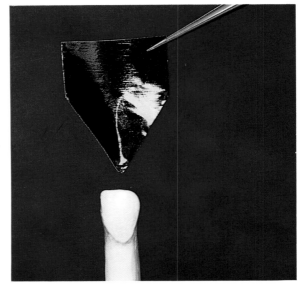

Fig. 6-18 The prepared platinum foil is shown in its relationship to the underlying die.

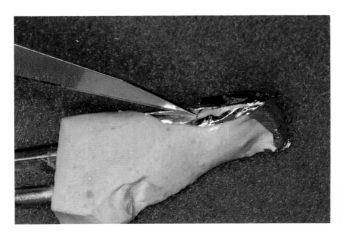

Fig. 6-19 Cut away the excess platinum foil beyond the cavosurface preparation line.

Fig. 6-20 Fold over the lateral aspects using fine-point tweezers. This is a progressive, wraparound procedure.

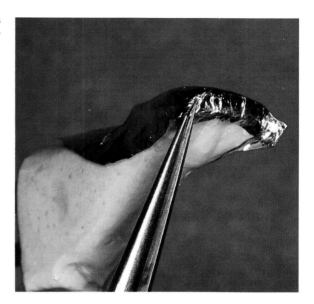

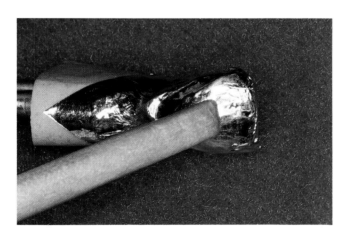

Fig. 6-21 Burnish the platinum foil onto the dies with an orangewood stick.

Fig. 6-22 Buccal and lingual views of the prepared platinum foil in position.

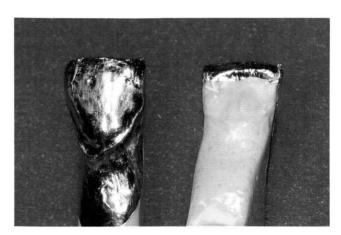

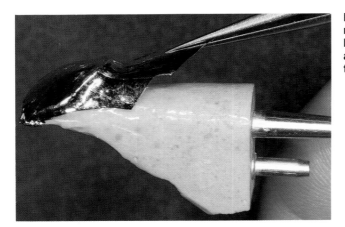

Fig. 6-23 Elevate the platinum foil off the underlying die by moving it from the cervical aspect and rotating it around the incisal edge.

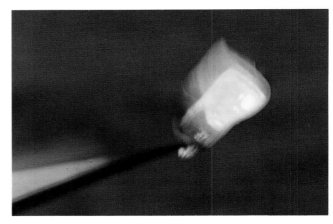

Fig. 6-24 Decontaminate the foil in a Bunsen burner. It should be heated until it glows orange.

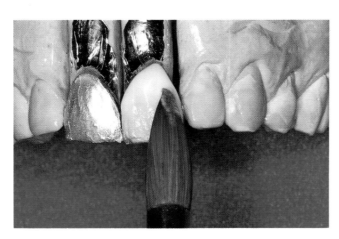

Fig. 6-25 The decontaminated foils are replaced on the dies and the matte color can be seen. The first wet slurry of porcelain is applied to the foil.

Fig. 6-26 Lift the foil and overlying initial porcelain off the die.

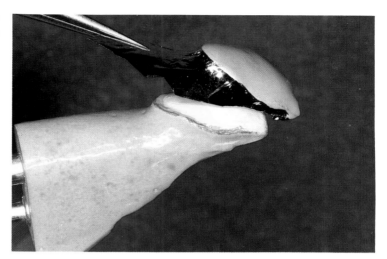

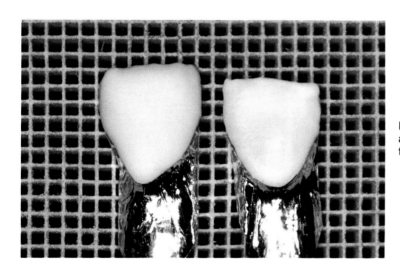

Fig. 6-27 The two foils and first application of porcelain are ready to be fired on a saggar tray.

Fig. 6-28 After the first firing, the laminate is built up to full contour utilizing the four-stage buildup: gingival third, cervical, body, and incisal porcelains.

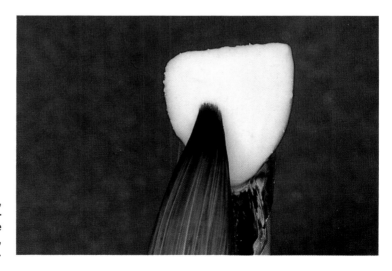

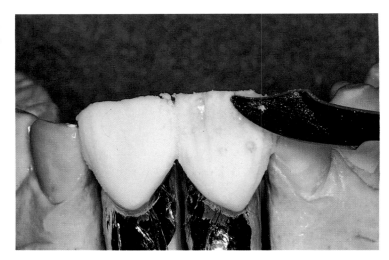

Fig. 6-29 The incisal porcelain can be cut back somewhat to lay in the special illusionary effects of translucency.

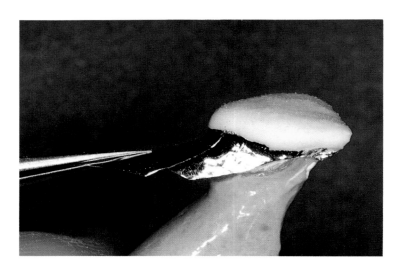

Fig. 6-30 Lift the foil and the completed porcelain buildup off the underlying die.

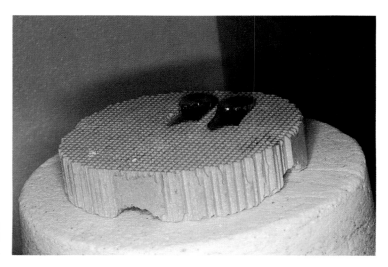

Fig. 6-31 The two laminate buildups are ready to be placed into the furnace.

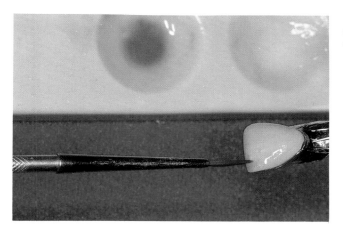

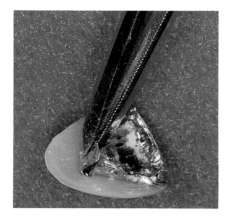

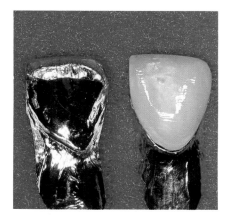

Fig. 6-32 The laminates can be characterized utilizing surface staining.

Fig. 6-33 Buccal and lingual views of the completed laminates showing the ongoing maintenance of the platinum foil form.

Fig. 6-34 Remove the platinum foil by teasing it away from the porcelain using fine-pointed tweezers. This may be facilitated by doing it under water.

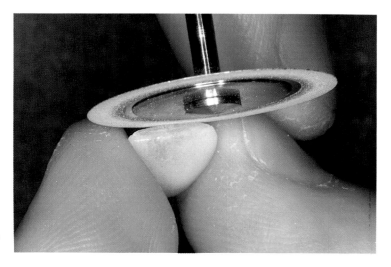

Fig. 6-35 Trim and refine the laminate margins.

4. Removal of Foil

By grasping the edge of the foil with the fine serrated-tip tweezers, gently pull the foil away from the veneer. Submerging the veneer in water will reduce surface tension for easier removal of foil. Lastly, the interface of the veneer is ready to be etched.

When the foil is peeled away from the interface of the finished veneer, the interface will have a smooth, glaze-like surface, not suitable for bonding. Therefore, it is advantageous to use a porcelain with optimum etching characteristics in order to develop an internal surface that will bond effectively to the tooth.

Porcelain Application

Because the porcelain buildup for a veneer averages 0.5 to 0.8 mm, the mix will dry very rapidly while working. Therefore, water and a liquid additive, or a special liquid medium, should be used to prevent this loss of moisture from the porcelain mix while buildup of the veneer is in progress. The porcelain should be condensed after the veneer is built to its final stage.

Buildup of porcelain veneers, especially on refractory investment, may take two or three applications before the desired form is obtained. If using the refractory technique (as opposed to the foil technique), manufacturers suggest that the refractory die be placed in distilled water for four or five minutes before each porcelain application.

The first application of porcelain should be 0.3 to 0.4 mm thick. Shrinkage and fissures are to be expected following firing with this thin, initial application. The second application of porcelain will cover any inaccuracies of the first and should be built to full contour. After condensing, fire the porcelain at the specified porcelain firing cycle and then glaze.

The esthetic results of the finished veneer are enhanced if the porcelain mix is applied in four stages to *(1)* the gingival third, *(2)* body, *(3)* incisal and *(4)* enamel shading (buildup). Mix the porcelain to a paste-like consistency for ideal stacking and firing results. Porcelain that is one shade darker than the overall prescribed shade should be applied to the gingival third. Then apply the prescribed shade of body porcelain from the gingival to the middle third and feather it to the incisal edge. If a mamelon effect is desired, three lobes of body porcelain can be scalped at the incisal aspect of the labial contour. The incisal porcelain is then applied to the desired length and should account for one quarter to one third of the incisal buildup. The remaining incisal buildup, and its extension over the incisal edge, is achieved by applying a thin layer of enamel porcelain over the entire incisal third. The porcelain should be condensed and contoured to its desired shape and then allowed to bench set for five minutes before firing.

Finishing and Contouring

Porcelain veneers should be finished with a high-speed (approximately 150,000 rpm) handpiece and microfine (15 to 45 grit size) friction-grip diamonds. Do not use larger grit sizes as they tend to chip the fragile porcelain laminate. Diamonds, when finishing with a low-speed (45,000 rpm) handpiece, do not build up the surface heat that a metal bur or stones would create. Contour facial areas using a flame-shaped diamond. Marginal areas of the veneer are lightly contoured with (carborundum) sandpaper disks.

If separating embrasures between veneers on a refractory model, use an ultrathin diamond disk (see Fig. 6-7) followed by a double-sided cutting disk to carefully reduce the refractory material at the gingival areas (see Fig. 6-8). Finish the incisal edges with a sandpaper disk, and redefine facial anatomy with a fine diamond contouring bur. Removal of as much refractory material as possible is important to reduce the amount of any residual ammoniated gasses during subsequent firing during glazing.

Glazing

A thin layer of porcelain-fusing glaze (1,700°F/927°C) is painted on the porcelain surface to seal any microporosities and achieve a more natural luster. To add chroma to the veneers, stains are applied—usually to the incisal or gingival third—

in areas requiring characteristic color (see Fig. 6-32). Paint a slurry mix of glaze over the labial surface, apply stains, and allow them to dry. The veneer is then fired to the desired surface glaze.

Adjustment and Placement on Master Model

In the foil technique, if all the previous steps are correctly performed, adjustment to the master cast or working model should be a minimal finishing procedure.

In the refractory technique, ready the second master cast utilizing a no. 1 round bur to trim below the gingival margin and to relieve embrasure obstructions to permit fitting of the fired veneers.

In the case of multiple veneers (whether platinum foil or refractory methods were used), a central incisor veneer is first placed on the master cast and the fit is checked. A medium-grit carborundum paper disk or extra-fine-grit diamond can be used to make any adjustments to allow for intimate fit. Remove this first veneer and place the adjacent veneer, making any necessary adjustments as before.

Once all veneers have been individually fitted to the master cast, use an ultrathin blade or medium coarse abrasive strip to relieve the contact area on the cast to the height of the interdental papillae. The two veneers are now reseated and contacts checked by pulling ultra-fine articulating paper through the contact area to mark any areas that bind. Gently mark and disk-trim both veneers until they are completely seated. The marking paper should be able to just pass passively through the contacts. Repeat the adjustment procedure moving progressively distally in the arch until all units are fitted.

Etching

Several methods and materials exist for etching the interface or inner aspect of the porcelain veneer. A safe, predictable, and time efficient system has been developed.

Place the labial surface of the veneer on a clay strip, allowing the concave inner aspect of the veneer to act as a receptacle. Then fill the interface of the veneer with the etching gel (e.g., 7.5% hydrofluoric acid) and allow it to stand for seven to ten minutes. The gel must occasionally be brushed up to the margins to ensure etching in this critical area (Fig. 6-36). Different porcelain

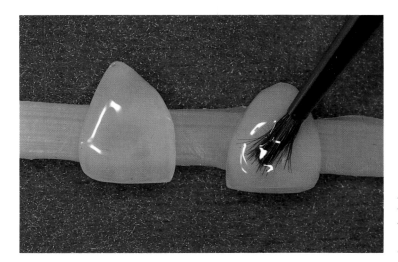

Fig. 6-36 Place the acid-etching medium within the concavity of the inner surface of the laminate. This must be gently agitated every few minutes and constantly brushed up toward the periphery of the laminate.

systems require different etching times with various etching mediums. Individual manufacturer's instructions must be followed for optimum results.

When the etching phase is completed, lift the entire clay strip by both edges and completely submerge the veneers in a 10% solution of baking soda and water until the acid is neutralized (Fig. 6-37). The gel will bubble and rise to the surface of the solution. Remove the veneer from the solution and dry.

Using 50 μm aluminum oxide particles at 20 psi

air pressure, air abrade the interface until it is free of etched ceramic debris. Clean the veneers in a detergent solution in an ultrasonic bath for three minutes each and dry with an oil-free air syringe or a jet of warm air. The complete veneers are now ready for bonding (Figs. 6-38 and 6-39). There is some evidence to indicate that these dried veneers should be placed in a furnace at 1,110°F (600°C) for five minutes to ensure complete drying and deactivation of the hydrofluoric acid.

Fig. 6-37 Neutralize the acid within a solution of bicarbonate of soda. The process is completed when the bubbling stops.

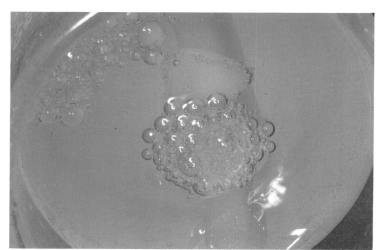

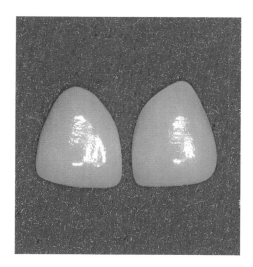

Fig. 6-38 Labial view of two completed laminates.

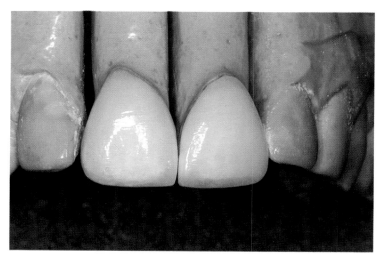

Fig. 6-39 The two laminates in position on the master cast.

Bibliography

Adar, P. Personal communication.

Asmussen, E. Adhaesiv reparation af porcelaen. Tandlaegebladet 83:352, 1979.

Bakir, N., Lautenschlager, E.P., and Greener, E.H. Curing of dental composites with visible lights. J. Dent. Res. 64(Spec. Issue; IADR/AADR Abstr. no. 608):242, 1985.

Barreto, M.T., and Bottaro, B.F. A practical approach to porcelain repair. J. Prosthet. Dent. 48:349, 1982.

Black, J.B. Esthetic restoration of tetracycline-stained teeth. J. Am. Dent. Assoc. 104:846, 1982.

Boksman, L., et al. Etched porcelain labial veneers. Ont. Dent. 62(1):13–19, 1985.

Bowen, R.L. Development of a silica-resin direct filling material. Report 6333. Washington: National Bureau of Standards, 1958.

Bowen, R.L. Properties of a silica-reinforced polymer for dental restorations. J. Am. Dent. Assoc. 66:57–64, 1963.

Boyer, D.B., and Chalkley, Y. Bonding between acrylic laminates and composite resin. J. Dent. Res. 61:489–492, 1982.

Brudevold, F., Gardner, D.E., and Smith, F.A. The distribution of fluoride in human enamel. J. Dent. Res. 35:420, 1956.

Buonocore, M.G.A. The Use of Adhesives in Dentistry. Springfield, Ill.: Charles C Thomas Publ. Co., 1975.

Buonocore, M.G.A. Simple method of increasing the adhesion of acrylic filling materials to enamel surfaces. J. Dent. Res. 34:849–53, 1955.

Calamia, J.R. Etched porcelain veneers: the current state of the art. Quintessence Int. 16:5–12, 1985.

Calamia, J.R. Etched porcelain facial veneers: a new treatment modality. N.Y. J. Dent. 53:255–259, 1983.

Calamia, J.R., and Simonsen, R.J. Effect of coupling agents on bond strength of etched porcelain. J. Dent. Res. 63:162–362, 1984.

Calamia, J.R., et al. Shear bond strength of etched porcelains. J. Dent. Res. 64(Spec. Issue; IADR/AADR Abstr. no. 1096):296, 1985.

Chering, W.S., Pulver, F., and Smith, D.C. Custom-made veneers for permanent anterior teeth. J. Am. Dent. Assoc. 105:1015, 1982.

Christiansen, G.J. Personal communication.

Christiansen, G.J. Veneering of teeth. State of the art. Dent. Clin. North Am. 29(2):373–391, 1985.

Christiansen, G.J. Veneers: state of the art. Oral presentation at American Academy of Esthetic Dentistry, Maui, Hawaii, August 1983.

Christiansen, G.J. Comparison of veneer types. Clinical Research Associates Newsletter. Provo, Utah. 10(4), 1986.

Eames, W.B., and Rogers, L.B. Porcelain repairs: retention after one year. Oper. Dent. 4:75–77, 1979.

Faunce, F.R. Method and apparatus for restoring badly discolored, fractured or cariously involved teeth. United States Patent Number: 3,986,261. Filed Dec. 5, 1973. Date of Patent: Oct. 19, 1976.

Faunce, F.R. Tooth restoration with preformed laminated veneers. Dent. Surv. 53(1):30, 1977.

Faunce, F.R., and Myers, D.R. Laminate veneer restoration of permanent incisors. J. Am. Dent. Assoc. 93(4):790–792, 1976.

Glantz, P. On wettability and adhesiveness. Odont. Revy 23(Suppl. 17):1, 1969.

Goldstein, R. Change Your Smile. Chicago: Quintessence Publ. Co., 1984.

Gratton, D.R., Jordan, R.E., and Teteruck, W.R. Resin bonded bridges: the state of the art. Ont. Dent. 60(5): 9–19, 1983.

Greggs, T.S. Method for cosmetic restoration of anterior teeth. United States Patent Number: 4,473,353. Filed Apr. 15, 1983. Date of Patent: Sept. 25, 1984.

Greggs, T.S. Personal communication.

Gwinnett, A.J., and Matsui, A. A study of enamel adhesives: the physical relationship between enamel and adhesive. Arch. Oral Biol. 12:1615, 1967.

Heyde, J.B., and Cammarato, V.T. The laminate veneers. Dent. Clin. North Am. 252:337–345, 1981.

Highton, R.M., Caputo, A.A., and Matyas, J. Effectiveness of porcelain repair systems. J. Prosthet. Dent. 42:292, 1979.

Hobo, S., and Iwata, T. A new laminate veneer technique using a castable apatite ceramic material. II. Practical procedures. Quintessence Int. 8:509–517, 1985.

Horn, H.R. Porcelain laminate veneers bonded to etched enamel. Dent. Clin. North Am. 27:671–684, 1983.

Horn, H.R. A new lamination: porcelain bonded to enamel. N.Y. State Dent. J. 49(6):401–403, 1983.

Hsu, C.S., Stangel, I., and Nathansen, D. Shear bond strength of resin to etched porcelain. J. Dent. Res. 64(Spec. Issue; IADR/AADR Abstr. no. 1095)296, 1985.

Hussain, M.A., Bradford, E.W., and Charlton, G. Effect of etching on the strength of a luminous porcelain jacket crown. Br. Dent. J. 147:89, 1979.

Ibsen, R.L. Personal communication.

Ibsen, R.L., and Strassler, H.E. An innovative method for fixed anterior tooth replacement utilizing porcelain veneers. Quintessence Int. 17:455, 1986.

Johnson, R.G. A new method for direct bonding orthodontic attachments to porcelain teeth using a silane coupling agent: an in vitro evaluation. Am. J. Orthod. 77:233, 1980.

Jordon, R.E., et al. Temporary fixed partial dentures fabricated by means of the acid-etch resin technique: a report of 86 cases followed up to three years. J. Am. Dent. Assoc. 96:994–1001, 1978.

Livaditis, G.J. Personal communication.

Livaditis, G.J. Cast metal resin-bonded retainers for posterior teeth. J. Am. Dent. Assoc. 101:926–929, 1980.

Livaditis, G.J. Resin bonded restorations: a clinical study. Int. J. Periodont. Rest. Dent. 1(4):71–79, 1981.

Livaditis, G.J., and Thompson, V.P. Etched castings: an improved retentive mechanism for resin-bonded retainers. J. Prosthet. Dent. 47:52–58, 1982.

Livaditis, G.J., Thompson, V.P., and Del Castillo, E. Resin bond to electrolytically etched nonprecious alloys for resin-bonded prostheses, abstract. J. Dent. Res. 60(Spec. Issue A):377, 1981.

McLaughlin, G. Porcelain fused to tooth—a new esthetic and reconstructive modality. Compend. Cont. Educ. Dent. 5(5):430–435, 1985.

McLaughlin, G. The etched metal bridge: a new laboratory technique. Dent. Lab. Rev. 57(3):32–34, 1982.

Myerson, R.L. Effects of silane bonding of acrylic resins to porcelain on porcelain structure. J. Am. Dent. Assoc. 78:113, 1969.

Newburg, R., and Pameijer, C.H. Composite resin bonded to porcelain with silane solution. J. Am. Dent. Assoc. 96:288–291, 1978.

Nixon, R.L. Bonding technique for porcelain veneers. The Forum of Esthetic Dentistry 3(8):1–11, 1985.

Nixon, R.L. Personal communication.

Nixon, R.L. Use of porcelain laminate veneers enhances foreshortened, worn teeth. Dentistry Today October 1984, pp. 27–31.

Nixon, R.L. The Chairside Manual for Porcelain Bonding. Wilmington, Del.: B.A. Videographics, 1987.

Nowlin, T.P., Barghi, N., and Norling, B.K. Evaluation of the bonding of three porcelain repair systems. J. Prosthet. Dent. 46:516–518, 1981.

Pincus, C.R. Building mouth personality. J. Calif. S. Dent. Assoc. 14:125–129, 1938.

Pincus, C.R. Building mouth personality. Alpha Omegan 42:163–166, 1948.

Pincus, C.R. Personal communication.

Pollack, B.R., and Blitzer, M.H. Esthetic veneering: material and techniques. Gen. Dent. 31:483–488, 1983.

Richter, W.A., and Ueno, H. Relationship of crown margin placement to gingival inflammation. J. Prosthet. Dent. 30:156, 1973.

Rochette, A.L. A ceramic bonded by etched enamel and resin for fractured incisors. J. Prosthet. Dent. 33:287–293, 1975.

Rochette, A.L. Attachment of a splint to enamel of lower anterior teeth. J. Prosthet. Dent. 30:418–423, 1973.

Ronk, S.L. Dental laminates: which technique? J. Am. Dent. Assoc. 102:186, 1981.

Ronk, S.L. Dental lamination: clinical problems and solutions. J. Am. Dent. Assoc. 104:844, 1982.

Silverstone, L.M., and Dogon, I.L. Proceedings of an International Symposium on the Acid Etch Technique. St. Paul, Minn.: North Central Publishing Co., 1975.

Simonsen, R.J. Clinical Applications of the Acid Etch Technique. Chicago: Quintessence Publ. Co., 1978.

Simonsen, R.J., and Calamia, J.R. Tensile bond strength of etched porcelain. J. Dent. Res. 61:297(Abstr. no. 1154), 1983.

Simonsen, R.J., Thompson, V.P., and Barrack, G. Etched Cast Restorations: Clinical and Laboratory Techniques. Chicago: Quintessence Publ. Co., 1983.

Strassler, H.E., and Buchness, G.F. Etched porcelain veneers: our newest cosmetic dentistry treatment modality. BCDS Forum. 5(2):7–9, 1985.

Vaidyanthan, J., et al. Film thickness and water sorption of composite cements. J. Dent. Res. 64(Spec. Issue; IADR/AADR Abstr. no. 45):179, 1985.

Visible-Curing Lights—Extra-Wide Area of Cure. Clinical Research Associates Newsletter. Provo, Utah. 8:1, 1984.

Special Effects and Characterization

Pinhas Adar

As previously discussed in this book, porcelain laminates were essentially developed to satisfy several different needs:

1. To replace missing parts of teeth, as in fractures

2. To esthetically improve discolored teeth

3. To create the illusion of better aligned teeth when teeth are malpositioned

4. To close spaces between teeth

Each of these individual situations requires a specific understanding of the nature of the porcelain and of the particular laboratory techniques used to overcome some of the inherent inadequacies in porcelain laminates. Closing diastemata requires a completely different buildup technique than does changing the color of a dark, unattractive tooth or replacing a missing incisal half of a fractured tooth.

Almost any porcelain can be baked and etched for a laminate veneer. Some manufacturers have specifically developed porcelains for this procedure. Their frit formulations are such that the veneer will supposedly etch in a more retentive pattern for better bond strength to enamel. The formulations also have increased amounts of opacifiers and metallic oxide pigments so that even in the 0.5 mm thickness of a laminate, intricate characterization and color effects can be developed.

Ceramic Buildup for Discolored Teeth

Tooth discoloration associated with childhood tetracycline ingestion can range from a yellow-brown through to a gray-blue-black stain. In these situations, within the laminate thickness limitations of 0.5 to 0.7 mm, *it is necessary to neutralize the underlying color and then create the illusion of normal tooth color and form.* It has been suggested that the composite resin luting agent should act as the primary opacifier, with a laminate of normal opacity to cover this discoloration. It is, however, more effective to have the opaquing incorporated into the porcelain veneer itself and utilize the composite resin luting agent only as an adjunct if needed. Opaquing the laminate makes it impossible for the dentist to add underlying composite resin tints and characterization to develop any additional special effects, because the overlying porcelain will be so opaque that the composite resin will not be visible through it.

There are several systems for opaquing dark stains. In some, there is an opaque powder provided just for this specific purpose. It can be used in the conventional manner of laying down a thin layer of opaque porcelain to neutralize the underlying tooth color and then building the tooth form over this. However, this procedure is inordinately difficult because of the sparsity of available space.

This system also requires a laminate about 1.2 mm thick, which means greater tooth reduction in preparation or more contour to the final restoration. If overcontouring is contraindicated, it is essential to prepare more than 1 mm of labial tooth surface. With this available space it is possible for a layer of opaque to be laid down first, followed by the normal buildup of porcelain.

Ironically, the deeper into the tooth that a bur cuts, the darker the underlying color appears to become, because it is the dentin which is discolored and the enamel being removed has usually masked some of this color. There is also a problem as dentinal tubules are exposed where enamel is removed, leaving only a narrow periphery or band of enamel to seal the overlying restoration to the tooth. This type of aggressive preparation is contraindicated in laminates and is contrary to the entire concept.

The following method is a variation on opaquing methods that is useful in neutralizing the dark underlying color while still providing lifelike color to the porcelain veneer.

It is possible to mix the same opaque porcelain powder with a dentin shade and create a mix of opacious dentin to be used as a body mask in the initial layer. This will allow penetration of some underlying color to the surface to (1) develop the illusion of color depth, and (2) reflect light back off the opaque particles in the mix to the surface. The three porcelain blends of cervical, body, and incisal ceramic are layered on top of this to the full contour of the tooth. A veneer in excess of 1 mm is still required to effectively neutralize the underlying tooth and produce an esthetic, natural-looking restoration with color depth and vitality.

The P.A. Opacity System

This alternative method—a layering technique—was developed by Willi Geller, M.D.C., in Zurich for the buildup of conventional crown-and-bridge restorations. In this technique, the dentin porcelains are blended with a white stain powder from the conventional staining kit. This blend can in turn be further modified by using other tints from the same system, such as orange to opaque and characterize the cervical region.

The mixture is applied in a very thin layer over the platinum foil matrix (Figs. 7-1 and 7-2). After firing this initial specially formulated layer, the subsequent layers are built up in the three dimensional system of cervical, body, and incisal porcelains. The mixing of the white tint or stain into the dentin porcelain allows the ceramist to neutralize the underlying darkly stained tooth. The neutralization can be complete because the white is effectively totally opaque. The degree of opacity can be modified by increasing the ratio of white to dentin porcelain in the mixture. The greater the proportion of white, the more opaque this initial layer will be. It is useful, however, not to completely neutralize the tooth but to allow some of the underlying color to selectively bleed through, thus providing the illusion of depth to the final veneer.

This layering technique is readily usable with any ceramic veneer system because any body shade can be blended with any of the commercially available white stains or tint kits.

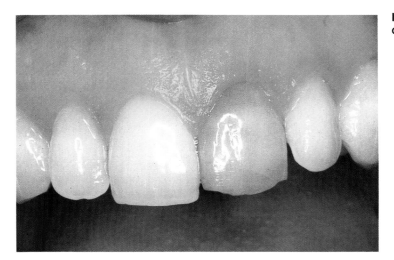

Fig. 7-1 Patient with a discolored central incisor.

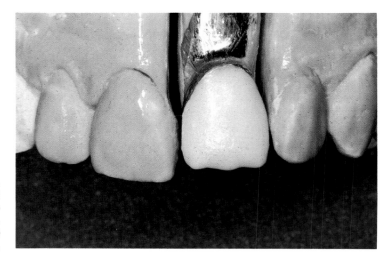

Fig. 7-2 A thin layer of "P.A. opacity" is applied to platinum foil. White stain pigment and dentin porcelain powder are mixed, and this layer is fired prior to body buildup.

The Creation of a Root Surface

It is a fallacious concept that to create the illusion of a root surface all that is required is to scribe a cementoenamel junction and then color the root area apical to it with an orange tint. In fact, that area beyond the cementoenamel junction—the root—has to be developed separately from the crown. This is because its underlying porcelain structure needs to contain considerably more opacious dentin.

Cervical Effects

Cervical areas should be decided upon beforehand so that the technician can first build up this portion of the laminate with the required increased opacity.

In the cervical or root area the opacious dentin will be laid down and then feathered out toward the cementoenamel junction. Over this, the technician will begin to build up the entire form of the laminate or tooth in dentin porcelain (Figs. 7-3 and 7-4). Once it is completed, a cutback is performed to lay in the enamel porcelain. This cutback begins at the incisal edge and is in turn feathered out toward the middle of the tooth (Fig. 7-5).

This three-stage buildup of body or dentin porcelain, cervical porcelain, and enamel porcelain is critical not only to the ultimate form of the tooth

Fig. 7-3 Cervical blend porcelain is applied to the apical one third of the laminate, blending into the middle or body one third.

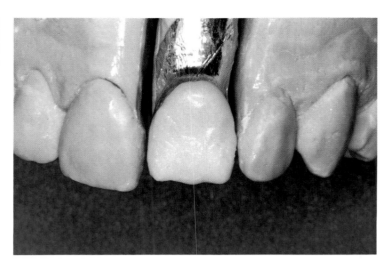

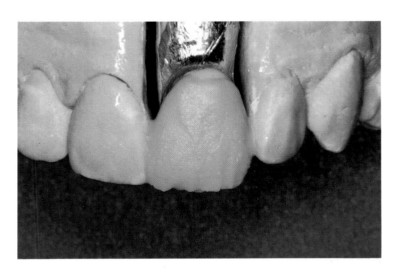

Fig. 7-4 Conventional buildup of body porcelain to full contour over a fired layer of P.A. opacity.

Fig. 7-5 The buildup is cut back to develop incisal porcelain effects.

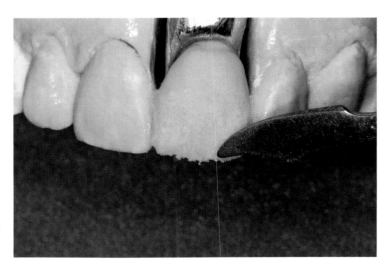

but also to the way the color will blend in harmoniously from the cervical area through to the incisal area. It is important for the technician to realize that all these layers must be built in *before firing,* because it is contraindicated to grind back the porcelain following baking. To do so will increase the risk of contaminating the porcelain or fracturing it in an attempt to create the space in the fired porcelain for these special color effects.

Incisal Effects

The incisal illusion is created by the following method. Three mixes of porcelain are made up:

1. Pure incisal porcelain

2. Pure translucent or clear porcelain

3. A 50:50 mixture of incisal and clear porcelains

The cutback should simulate anatomical tooth form and the way dentin is laid down in the three mamelons. The incisal porcelain is now laid down in sequential "piano key" striations from the mesial and the distal edges of the tooth to form the palatal aspect of the incisal edge of the remaining dentin (Figs. 7-6 and 7-7). These "piano keys" start sequentially at the mesial and distal aspects of the tooth with a "key" of pure incisal blend porcelain. Too much clear porcelain in these areas will create an area of "black color," because the darkness from the back of the mouth is transmitted through the clear porcelain. The periphery is first built of pure incisal blend, the adjacent key is a mixture of incisal and clear porcelain, and the following "piano key" or finger-like extension is of pure clear porcelain. Thereafter, the same three blends are sequentially laid down until they meet in the center. These projections should be laid down to the

Fig. 7-6 The labial aspect of the incisal edge is built up in sequential "piano keys" of clear, incisal, and clear-incisal porcelain blends. This forms the base for laying down internal characterization staining effects.

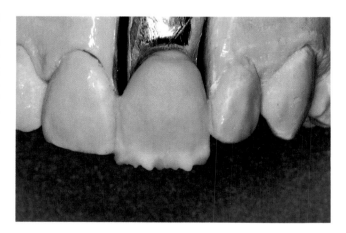

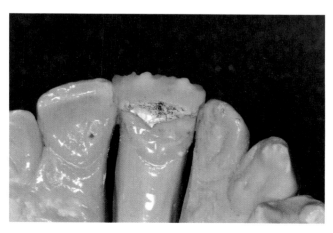

Fig. 7-7 Palatoincisal view of Fig. 7-6.

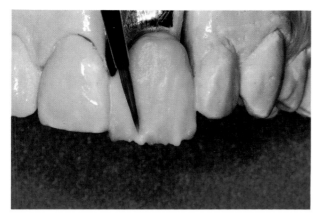

Fig. 7-8 Violet stain is layered in to develop the illusion of translucency.

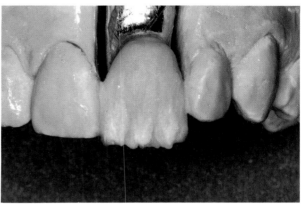

Fig. 7-9 Milky-white stain and yellow-orange color are layered-in to develop a mamelon effect contrasting with the violet translucency.

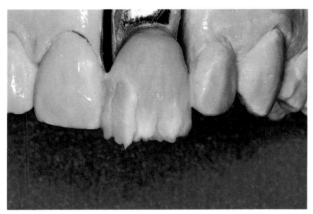

Fig. 7-10 Internal characterization is overlaid with the same three incisal mixtures of porcelain using the same piano key format to develop the illusion of depth.

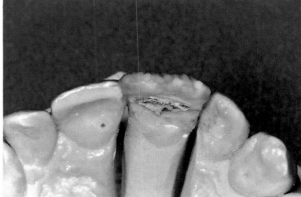

Fig. 7-11 Palatoincisal view of the completed buildup.

desired length of the tooth. *The porcelain must be considerably more moist than normal,* as in such thin sections it tends to dry out rapidly.

To create the illusion of deep translucency, the color violet is inlaid on the periphery—mesially and distally—and then in between the mamelons (Fig. 7-8). The mamelons themselves are now inlaid and highlighted by mixing a milky white porcelain with either yellow or orange stain (Fig. 7-9). To create the illusion of greater contrast between the various inlaid colors, the orange and the violet layers are separated by the thin milky white line. This serves not so much to demarcate the colors but to emphasize each one respectively. This incisal edge porcelain is now overlaid in much the same way, with pure incisal porcelain on the mesial and distal surfaces, and the pure clear porcelain over the areas where the violet stain is inlaid between the mamelons. This allows the violet to show through to the surface, but from within (Fig. 7-10).

Depending on the effect desired, the veneer can be overlaid with pure clear porcelain to increase the illusion of depth superimposed upon the underlying stains, or it may be toned down by overlaying the mixture of clear and incisal porcelains.

The final shape of the veneer from the cervical margin to the incisal edge is completed by placing a thin layer of the incisal/clear mixture across the complete surface of the laminate (Fig. 7-11).

Creating the "Halo" Effect at the Incisal Edge

A "halo" is created by mixing dentin porcelain with white stain and framing the entire incisal complex with this mixture all the way from the mesial aspect across the incisal edge and up the distal aspect of the tooth (Fig. 7-12). The halo framing the tooth will serve in turn to highlight all internal aspects within this frame. It adds contrast to all aspects of the tooth within its boundaries by ending at a well defined incisal edge instead of blending out with translucency. This halo serves the important purpose of emphasizing all the previous special effects that have been created.

The incisal treatment will obviously vary in the older patient, because of the usual ongoing abrasion of the incisal edge of the tooth and the underlying dentin coming to the surface. This effect will necessitate laying in a mixture of orange-brown color closer to the incisal edge surface. The final laminate can be seen in Fig. 7-13.

Fractured Teeth (Class IV Fractures)

The problem with creating a porcelain laminate for a Class IV fractured incisor, when the entire

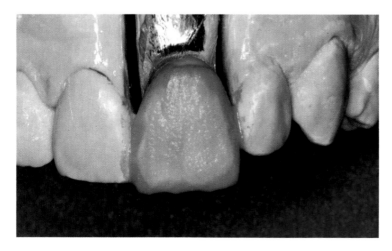

Fig. 7-12 The incisal halo effect is developed.

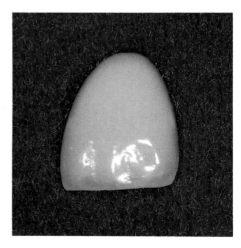

Fig. 7-13 The laminate is ready for insertion.

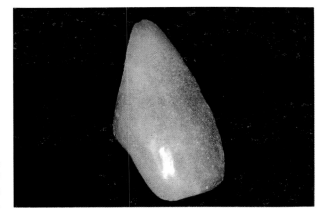

Fig. 7-14 The P.A. opacity is developed in the region of fracture unsupported by the tooth.

incisal edge or a portion thereof is missing, is in creating sufficient opacity in the region where the laminate is to be unsupported by the underlying tooth and dentin (Fig. 7-14). If this region is not opaqued but is simply built up in the conventional manner, it will show up as a gray-black area. This grayness will in fact be the darkness from the back of the mouth that is not being blocked by the opaque and is reflecting through the translucent laminate. In this situation, the layer technique of Geller can be utilized again to develop natural tooth color in the unsupported porcelain. The laminate will replace the fracture and be blended back with increasing translucency to allow the natural tooth to become an integral part and background color for the whole restoration. It is important for the technician to realize that the original tooth cannot be recreated exactly, but that the goal is to create an illusion to fool the human eye.

Esthetics are very much "in the eye of the beholder." This subjective opinion is influenced by the lay press and consumer fads. It will vary from country to country and even within certain social groups of one country. The idea of the white "piano keys" effect of the so-called "Hollywood smile" may well be the desire of some sectors of the American population, and this effect can be readily obtained with porcelain laminates. However, it is incumbent upon the technician to learn both the science of the ceramic system and develop artistic abilities so that when called upon, he or she can mimic nature in the course of doing a single restoration that will match the adjacent tooth in every detail or imperfection. These imperfections may well be what that particular patient considers to be natural looking.

Bibliography

Christensen, G.J. Comparison of veneer types. Clinical Research Associates Newsletter. Provo, Utah. 10(4): 1–2, 1986.

Geller, W. Personal communication, 1979.

Goldstein, R.E. Esthetics in Dentistry. Philadelphia: J.B. Lippincott, 1976.

Indigo, B. Personal communication, 1978.

Materdomini, D. Personal communication, 1987.

Nixon, R.L. The Chairside Manual for Porcelain Bonding. Wilmington, Del.: B.A. Videographics, 1987.

Placement of Veneers

8

The Three-Stage Porcelain Veneer Try-In

Prior to the final luting of the porcelain veneers, it is important to go through a try-in stage, which is a three-phase process:

1. The intimate adaptation of each individual porcelain laminate to the prepared tooth surface must be checked.

2. The collective fit and relationship of one laminate to another and the contact points need to be evaluated.

3. The color needs to be assessed and, if necessary, modified.

Preliminary Procedures

The teeth should be isolated with a cheek retractor (Clearview, L.D. Caulk, Milford, Del.). If there are temporary veneers in position, they should be peeled away; if necessary, they can be cross hatched with a bur and split apart using a blunt-ended instrument (GCI Crown Remover, G.C. International Corp., Scottsdale, Ariz.), thus exposing the prepared enamel below.

If the finish line has been extended to or below the gingival margin, the soft tissues should be gently displaced with a thin gingival retraction cord prior to the try-in of the veneers.

The veneers will be returned from the laboratory in a protective box in their etched state. *These fragile veneers must be handled with utmost care.* In order to minimize contamination, they should be handled at their edges and on the unetched labial surface.

- The inner aspect of each veneer should be inspected to see that it is evenly etched and that the etch extends all the way to the marginal periphery. *A drop of water placed on a correctly etched surface will spread and wet it evenly,* indicative of an entire etch.
- Check the laminate periphery to see that it is smooth and then place the veneer on the cast to see that it covers the preparation entirely and that the fit is accurate.
- Check the laminate for crack lines and foreign body inclusions using the composite resin curing light as a transilluminator.

Stage 1: Check for Individual Fit

Clean the teeth with a slurry of fine flour of pumice that contains no oils or fluoride. A nonwebbed rubber cup is the rotary instrument of choice because a brush may injure the gingiva, causing hemorrhage and subsequent contamination of the etched surface. Clean the contact areas with a fine composite resin finishing strip. The patient should be in a supine or horizontal position so that the labial aspect of the teeth to be veneered can be made horizontal or parallel to the floor, to aid in preventing the veneers from sliding off.

Select the most distal veneer and try it in on the respective tooth. *If the veneer does not fit in position immediately, do not force it.* Check for any undercuts and contact point impingement and use a microfine (LVS no. 6) diamond under magnification to adjust it until it seats easily.

Then check the veneer margins on the prepared tooth for accuracy and intimacy of fit. A drop of glycerine placed on the etched surface can facilitate adhesion of the veneer to the tooth surface. Try in each of the laminates individually and check the margins.

Stage 2: Collective Fit Try-In

The interproximal contacts must now be confirmed by trying in all the laminates together. Adjust any contact that is too tight, using an LVS no. 6 diamond and the utmost care. All veneers should fit passively in place.

Stage 3: Color Check

The final color of the restoration is the combined result of several factors and not only the porcelain shade selected.

Factors That Influence Color

- The original tooth color
- The porcelain shade selected and amount of opacifier added
- The color and opacity of the composite resin luting agent
- The use of resin shade modifiers and characterizers behind the veneers and ceramic tints on the surface

These factors have varying influences on the colors. It is difficult to ascertain the actual color of a veneer placed on a tooth because there is a space between the enamel surface and the veneer itself. This "air refraction" prevents the underlying tooth color from being transmitted through to the surface of the veneer. The porcelain/tooth interface can be filled with a fluid, which will then transmit some of the underlying color to the porcelain. Glycerine, which is water soluble and readily removed with a water spray or ultrasonic cleaner, is an adequate light and color transmission medium. It has more viscosity than water and once cleaned will not interfere with the adhesion of the etched surface. The glycerine is also an excellent guide as to composite resin shade selection.

Place one laminate in position with glycerine and then compare it to the shade tab selected by the patient. If the laminate appears darker than the shade tab, then a lighter colored composite

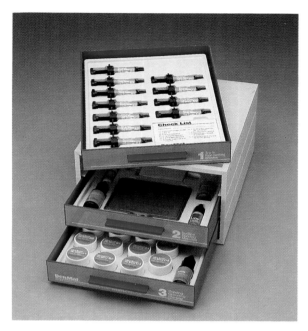

Fig. 8-1 A specially formulated and color-keyed try-in paste (Advanced Laminate Kit, Den-Mat Corp., Santa Maria, Calif.).

resin should be selected to modify the darkening effect of the underlying tooth. Conversely, if the laminate appears lighter than the shade tab, a darker composite resin is required. The next step is to utilize one of the color-keyed try-in pastes (e.g., Advanced Laminate Kit, Den-Mat Corp., Santa Maria, Calif.) to evaluate the patient's acceptance of the shade.

Composite Resin Color Check

The actual light-cured composite resin luting agent can be placed on the veneer next and the veneer reseated on the prepared tooth. The excess resin is removed with an explorer and the "final" color will become evident. If the patient is still unhappy, an adjacent veneer can be tried with a lighter or darker shade, and in this manner a shade check is done to ascertain the most esthetically pleasing color for the patient.

Caution must be used to avoid exposing the veneer and composite resin luting agent to the operating light, which may initiate the curing process. This cautionary measure is more critical with the "dual" cure type of composite resin, in which cure is initiated by white light and continues via a chemical cure process (Ultra Bond, Den-

Mat Corp., Santa Maria, Calif.; Heliolink, Vivadent, Tonawanda, N.Y.).

The basic shades in any of the commercial composite resin luting kits can usually be modified, enhanced, and characterized by some of the special kits of intense stains available. These same kits also provide opaquing systems that may be useful on some of the darkly stained teeth.

It is important to place a small portion of the selected composite resin on a white pad, cure it, and then compare its shade with an uncured portion. Many composite resins change color on initial curing, and it is prudent to be aware of this and to compensate for it before final seating of the laminate. In addition, most composite resin luting agents will undergo a further shift in color over the next 72 hours in the moist oral environment. This too can be checked by placing the cured sample of composite resin in a beaker of water for several days and comparing it to an uncured sample.

It has been suggested that one can try in the veneer with only the aid of water or glycerine, but this will unfortunately not allow for the influence of the interspersed composite resin affecting the shade of the laminate, although it would transmit the underlying color from the tooth. A better technique is to use the specially formulated and color-keyed try-in paste (Advanced Laminate Kit, Den-Mat Corp., Santa Maria, Calif.) (Fig. 8-1). Again, the final color is the result of four factors—the tooth, the porcelain, the composite resin, and the veneer itself—not just any two factors.

In assessing the relative impact of each of the four factors affecting the final shade, it is interesting to note that in many instances the actual shade of the porcelain has only nominal bearing on the bonded final veneer. This is because in most cases the laminate is only 0.5 mm thick and rather translucent. The underlying tooth color and the resin can modify its shade dramatically.

The available manufactured shade guides are not ideal for laminates. They are too thick and are made up of several different layers, including opaques. In addition, they are fabricated in quartz—not the porcelain used for laminates. The ideal is to have a ceramist make up a shade guide of porcelain laminates exactly as he or she would fabricate them, and then use these to select a shade.

Opaquing, Characterizing, and Staining

The laminate color should be inherent in the porcelain. However, because of its extreme thinness, the veneer can be characterized on its internal surface by the use of various composite resin color characterization kits. The veneer is etched and silanated and the colored resin is painted onto this etched surface. The veneers can then be tried in, and if the color is satisfactory the resin stain can be cured onto the veneers in very thin layers. Too great a thickness will impede proper placement. The veneers are then luted in position with the usual composite resin, which will not blend and smear the cured stains.

Veneers can also be characterized externally using a special laminate low-fusing stain system (Ceri-tint, Den-Mat Corp., Santa Maria, Calif.), which fuses at approximately 1,400°F (760°C), supposedly avoiding any laminate deformation. Alternatively, the laminate can be supported with an instant investment (Gresco Products, Inc., Stafford, Tex.), which when set facilitates staining with any conventional system.

Opaquing

The problem with opaquing is that the veneer color will need to be derived from less than 0.5 mm of material. Even a metal ceramic crown has about 1.2 mm or more of porcelain from which to develop color and opaque the metal.

Several methods have been advocated for opaquing the veneer. Some technicians advocate laying down striae of opaque porcelain as a base and building normally above this. The "P.A. opacity" system, using white stain, is another (see chapter 7). Most of the systems result in some loss of vitality for the veneer. It has also been advocated that the opacity be developed below the veneer by using a thicker layer of luting resin to neutralize the stained tooth. The apparent fallacy in this concept is that for the same thickness, porcelain can be made more opaque than the resin. In addition, the resin thickness in a well-fitting laminate should be in the realm of 60 μm. The added thickness of opaquing resin would weaken the final restoration because porcelain is a considerably stiffer material than resin. The large amount of resin also changes the characteristics of the three layered "sandwich" (i.e.,

tooth-resin-porcelain). The porcelain and tooth have similar coefficients of expansion and the usual thin layer of resin will not be greatly influenced by thermal changes. A larger dimension of resin will begin to show considerably larger dimensional changes with thermal activity, which will compromise the seal, retention, and strength of the veneer. The thicker layer of resin also increases the polymerization shrinkage factor. The added space taken by the resin would be better utilized by a comparable amount of porcelain.

Opaquing Localized Areas. Occasionally teeth are discolored in striae or localized small areas. If the surrounding tooth color is normal then these discreet areas can readily be opaqued with resin. It is extremely difficult for a technician to opaque only certain areas, particularly when not seeing the clinical patient. In these situations, once the laminate is returned from the laboratory, the dark area of the tooth should be selectively ground away. This will facilitate placement of extra opaque resin to neutralize the discolored area and bring it to a similar shade as the surrounding tooth substance. In general, always keep opaque away from the margins of a laminate because it will prevent the laminate from blending in with the rest of the tooth. *If increased thickness of resin is being used to facilitate opaquing, these areas should not be areas of heavy function.*

When the tooth is severely stained (e.g., by tetracycline) then it becomes essential to derive the final veneer color predominately from the porcelain itself. The resin may be used only to *help neutralize* the underlying shade of the discolored tooth. In extremely darkly stained teeth the laminate may not be sufficiently opaque, and to compensate, the resin may need to be highly opaque and may even need to be of additional thickness. This can be achieved in one of three ways:

1. By placing a die spacer of ± 0.1 mm on the actual die surface

2. By placing a spacer (e.g., calcium hydroxide liner) on the surface of the prepared tooth prior to impression taking

3. By trying on the laminate with the resin, and if it is still too dark, removing more tooth substance within the boundaries of the original preparation; this available space will be filled in by an increased amount of opaque resin

If shade modification does not need to be as extreme, the tooth, via the resin, can become an integral part of the final color. The resin chosen should not be opaque then; some of the underlying tooth color should be allowed to transmit through to the outer surface of the porcelain veneer.

The composite resin material used during the try-in phase will generally need to be removed entirely; this is done by placing the veneers in a container of pure alcohol in an ultrasonic cleaner for ten minutes. This removal can in fact be facilitated by the presence of glycerine on the etched surface of the laminate, if the glycerine was used to aid adhesion during the try-in phase to check fit and contact points. It is important to remove all this composite resin prior to the final process of luting. The color of the veneers at the try-in will be very similar but possibly not exactly the same as the final color, because of the ongoing changes that take place in composite resins during the total polymerization process. However, for the most part this color change will not be noticeable by anyone but the technician or dentist.

Luting Agents

Although both light-cured systems and chemically activated systems are available in the marketplace, the advantages offered by the light-cured system make it a considerably better choice. The fact that the system will cure only when exposed to light facilitates try-ins, modifications, and a color check with the chosen material prior to final seating. It also makes easy the removal of gross excess composite resin while it is still soft, prior to curing, and thus allows for easier final polishing and trimming of the margins.

There is a potential problem in the light-cured system in very opaque or thick veneers when insufficient light may be available to totally polymerize the luting material. *In these situations it is essential to use the dual cure system, in which a chemically cured process is initiated by light.*

The composite resin systems may be broadly classified as microfills, conventionals, and hybrids. Each category has its own particular advantages or disadvantages. It would appear that the "submicrofill hybrid" provides the best combination of favorable features. It has a film thick-

---

ness of 20 μm or less, relatively high compressive and tensile strengths, and low water absorption. The difference in particle size also provides for a slightly different optical refractive process and adequate polishability.

Once the three stage try-in has been completed, the veneers are ready for final placement.

Veneer Placement Procedure

1. Tissue Management

Place the patient in the supine or recumbant position. Retraction cords should be placed in the gingival sulcus to decrease the crevicular fluid flow, which would interfere with the adhesion and the seal between the laminate and the underlying enamel; they also displace the tissue to allow for direct visibility when placing and finishing veneers. All of these procedures—from try-in through final cementation—may be done with the aid of local anesthesia for finishing of the margins, which may be sulcular and may be somewhat uncomfortable.

2. Layout

The veneers have been tried in, checked, and modified, if necessary, so that the interproximal areas all fit passively. *It is important to realize that no modification for shape is done until the final seating and curing are completed.* Now lay out the cleaned, etched veneers in their respective

---

tooth order, in easy reach. All of the necessary instrumentation and materials should be assembled and laid out in the appropriate sequence of use. This will prevent any slowing down during the bonding procedure, which may result not only in loss of time but also in potential contamination of either the etched enamel or etched porcelain surfaces. The previously selected shade of composite resin with modifiers is also placed within easy proximity.

> **The bonding of the porcelain laminate to the tooth is in fact a series of links: etched enamel— to enamel/dentin bonding agent— to luting composite resin—to unfilled resin—to hydrolyzed silane—to etched porcelain (see Fig. 4-22).**

3. Silanation

First treat the etched surface of the veneers with the silane coupling agent to enhance the adhesive properties of the resin. The silane bond enhancer may be preactivated and hydrolyzed or it may need to be activated with an acid. A preactivated silane is painted onto the etched porcelain surface and allowed to dry for about one minute. The excess alcohol vehicle is then gently evaporated by passing a stream of air parallel to and approximately 6 in. above the surface of the laminate. This will leave a dry, silane-coated veneer. In the nonhydrolyzed form the surface of the laminate must first be conditioned with an acid medium to hydrolyze and activate the subsequent layer of silane. It is important to follow the particular manufacturer's instructions.

4. Enamel Activation

Clean the teeth with a slurry of fine pumice and water using a rubber cup and/or brush to remove all traces of salivary glycoproteins and previous composite resins from the try-in. If a brush is used it should not approach the gingiva, because it may induce hemorrhage. A nonwebbed rubber cap is preferable. The pumice should contain no fluoride or oils. Wash and air dry the teeth.

5. Isolation

Isolate the teeth with cheek retractors and cotton rolls. A 2-in.-square piece of gauze may be placed over the throat to further decrease moisture contamination. Use of a rubber dam would be ideal, but it is extremely difficult to use effectively; therefore, the above-mentioned system is reasonably adequate. Place a saliva ejector near the back of the throat and instruct the patient to breathe through his or her nose, further decreasing the moisture contamination that can be caused by humid vapor escaping the lungs.

6. Enamel Etching

The appropriate tooth is isolated on both sides by placing either mylar strips or a dead soft metal matrix band mesially and distally.

The tooth is etched with a 30% to 37% phosphoric acid solution for 15 to 20 seconds. The etchant must reach the very periphery of the preparation where a seal is highly critical to the long-term success of the restoration. Gingival displacement is important to expose this margin and prevent contamination. *The etching material (gel or liquid) is washed from the enamel surfaces with copious amounts of water for a full 30 seconds.* Liquid acid solutions wash off easier than gels, in which the methyl cellulose vehicle may be drawn into the etched enamel pores and remain there, acting as a contaminant and thus decreasing the bonding ability.

Do not let the patient rinse or in any way contaminate this etched enamel surface with saliva. If this occurs the surface must be re-etched for ten seconds, washed, and dried again to redevelop a reactive enamel surface. When washing, use high-speed evacuation to prevent the patient from tasting the acid, which may burn sensitive tissues. When changing the cotton rolls, be especially careful not to let the cheek or lip touch the tooth surface. The enamel surface is ideally dried with a stream of warm air (HandiDri, Den-Mat Corp., Santa Maria, Calif.) to ensure an uncontaminated, oil-free surface. This apppears to enhance bond strength by approximately 29%.[1] The air syringe on dental units may have the air lines contaminated with oil or water (this may be checked for by blowing on a wristwatch crystal or clean amalgam squeeze cloth). Remove the mylar strips and replace them with dead-soft metal matrix bands or the thinner (0.0005-in.) foil.

7. Application of Dental Bonding Agent

Again isolate the underlying etched tooth surface with matrix strips and coat it with a combined enamel-dental bonding agent of the light-activated type, which is gently air dispersed into a thin, even layer. *All excess bonding agent must be gently blown aside;* otherwise, it may pool and cure in these thick areas where there is no oxygen inhibition to prevent hardening. These hard nodules would pose a problem when trying to seat the laminate. Light cure this evenly dispersed layer to seal the tooth surface.

Next coat the internal aspect of the veneer (which has been silanated) with an unfilled resin bonding liquid; blow it into a thin layer but do not light cure it. Some manufacturers have combined the silane and resin bonding agent into one liquid (Ceriprime, Den-Mat Corp., Santa Maria, Calif.). Place the composite resin luting agent on the laminate, using some form of syringe and express the material into the center so that it spreads laterally, without trapping air bubbles.

8. Seating Sequence

It is best to seat one laminate at a time.

In multi-unit cases, start with the distal most tooth on each side of the arch and work mesially to the canine. Next seat the two central incisors simultaneously to ensure that they match. The two lateral incisors are then seated, one at a time, to accommodate any discrepancies in overall fit.

It is essential to move the unit light away from the operative field because it has the potential to start the autopolymerization process in any of these light activated materials.

Some clinicians feel that it is useful to take sticky wax and attach some form of handle (such as a toothpick) to the labial surface of the veneer, but others find it easier to manipulate the veneers without this accessory; it is, of course, a purely personal preference.

9. Placement

Rotate the veneer onto the buccal surface of the tooth and then gently manipulate it until contact is made in the region of the gingival finish line. The motion must be a gently rocking or "pulsing" motion that *slowly* allows the excess material to escape from all sides of the veneer. The gross excess may be removed with a firm, pointed paint-

brush or a curette. It is important *not to slide* the veneer into place. Passing it over the incisal edge may wipe the internal aspect of the veneer clean of the composite resin, leaving a void. This can be prevented by rotating it about the incisal edge into place.

Once the veneer is in place and seated, check the intimacy of fit between the margin and the preparation line with an explorer. Hold the laminate firmly in position to prevent "suck-back" and begin the polymerization process with the light. Cure for just 20 seconds from the lingual aspect and a further 20 seconds from the labial aspect in the incisal half of the tooth. Now remove the rest of the excess partially cured material—still holding the veneer tightly in place—from the gingival margin and interproximal area, using a sharp scaler and/or an explorer. The two matrix strips are now pulled from the buccal aspect toward the lingual aspect to clear the interproximal areas of excess material. **The matrix strips must be reinserted between the teeth to prevent them from bonding to one another.** The light is then reapplied to the labial and lingual surfaces of the veneer to complete the polymerization process.

During this curing process, it is essential to maintain complete stability of the relationship between the veneer and the underlying tooth. The polymerization process is completed by *curing the various areas of the veneer for at least two minutes each.* This extra time is important due to the fact that the light has to travel through the porcelain to reach the underlying composite resin.

The more excess resin that is removed prior to the finishing process, the easier the final finishing will be.

10. Curing

The white light systems for curing are remarkably effective, but the factors or variables involved in resin curing should be noted.

- **Time.** The greater the time the resin is exposed, the greater the percentage of cure.
- **Angle of contact.** The light should contact the resin at right angles to its surface—not at an oblique angle—for the maximum effectiveness.
- **Shade of the resin.** It appears that darker shades of resin and resins with increased opacifiers in them need an increased amount of time for curing.

- **Composite resin composition.** The exact formulation varies from resin to resin and within the specific categories of microfill through to the hybrids and macrofill types. There is also a variation in the degree of cure when exposed to the same amount of light.
- **Distance.** The distance of the light source to the surface of the composite resin should never be more than 1 mm.

In addition, one should note that the actual light source for the curing unit has an ever-decreasing intensity during its life-span and this should be checked routinely every month. In addition, those units that utilize a fiber optic cord show an ongoing decrease in their effectiveness because of constant bending and breakage of the fiber optic bundles associated with manipulation. These factors can be checked using an electric light monitor or using a ring of Teflon of standardized thickness. Composite resin is placed within this ring and exposed to the light, whereupon the ring is removed and the under surface of the composite resin checked to see if it is fully cured.

In general, curing of laminates is considerably more efficacious when using two lights—one from the buccal aspect and one from the lingual aspect. It would appear that the simultaneous use of two lights results in a deeper and more complete cure than the same degree of single exposure from either side.[2, 3]

In addition, it is also more useful to have the tip size on the light source to be somewhere between 12 to 15 mm in diameter in order to expose greater surfaces of the tooth to the curing process and to keep the tips in one position before moving on to expose another part of the laminate.

New advances include the use of a soft laser to more rapidly and fully cure the composite resin luting material thereby enhancing the ultimate strength of the veneers.[4]

11. Finishing

The finishing procedures are best accomplished with the aid of some form of ×2 to ×4 magnification. Following complete polymerization, chip off any excess composite resin with a carbide interproximal carver or gold foil knife. The four finishing instruments in the LVS kit are designed to correct any marginal discrepancies. First a carbide finishing bur with straight profile, such as the LVS no. 5 (Brasseler, Savannah, Ga.) should be gently inserted under the gingival margin. Using a copious water spray, run the instrument along the interface between the veneer and the underlying tooth surface to remove all excess resin. This should never be done dry because the heat generated will affect the composite resin luting agent. The carbide should remove the resin without scoring the remaining enamel or marring the porcelain. Once the resin is removed, check the margin to ensure that the laminate is a direct continuation of the remaining subgingival enamel. If it is not, use a microfine diamond point (LVS no. 7) to gently machine down the excess porcelain until the emergence profile of the enamel becomes confluent with that of the veneer (i.e., any horizontal ledge of porcelain beyond the enamel should be removed).

A polishing diamond (LVS no. 6 or no. 7) is used next to refine this interface of tooth/resin/porcelain. The polishing of the veneer is done with ceramic polishing points and then a diamond dust-impregnated paste with a nonwebbed rubber cup. Move the edge of the rubber cup up underneath the free gingival margin to bring the junction between the veneer, resin, and tooth to a high luster, ensuring that this area does not become a depository for microbial plaque. This final polishing can take five minutes or more per tooth. The interproximal areas should be cleared with the appropriate-grit Compostrip (Premier Dental Products, Norristown, Pa.) and polished with composite resin finishing strips. Check the interproximal contacts to see that floss passes through smoothly and does not catch or tear.

Lingual Finishing and Occlusal Equilibration. Finish the lingual aspect of the veneer/enamel interface with a football-shaped diamond (LVS no. 8) to remove excess resin. Evaluate the porcelain margin and, if necessary, refine it with the microfine diamond (15 μm size). Once again polish with the diamond dust on a rotating felt wheel and webbed rubber cup or a ceramic polishing wheel. The contact areas are cleaned with metal and then composite resin polishing strips and checked with dental floss.

12. Occlusal Assessment

The last step at the laminate placement appointment is to verify occlusion and ensure that the veneers do not make excessive contact with the opposing arch in any excursive movements of the mandible. This is obviously more critical when the incisal edge is lapped due to a fracture or the desire to increase the length of the teeth. If all the anterior teeth have been veneered to include the incisal edges, then a definitive occlusal relationship must be worked out. It would be ideal to distribute the load during mandibular excursive movements over as many teeth as possible, so that any one porcelain veneer extension is not responsible for withstanding the entire load. This decreases the potential for fracture of the laminate and excessive wear of the opposing arch. *A night guard is a useful adjunct to prevent these problems during sleep.*

13. Cosmetic Contouring

After several days (to ensure complete polymerization of the resin) the veneer can further be refined with fine diamonds for esthetic harmony. The bonded veneer is, at this stage, extremely strong and readily amenable to cosmetic contouring. ***The unsupported porcelain veneer should never be contoured until bonding is completed.*** The contouring is done with microfine (LVS no. 6 or no. 7) diamonds and finished with the porcelain polishing wheels and/or diamond polishing paste.

The final veneer provides the patient with the durability and beauty of porcelain, coupled with minimal tooth reduction and dentin exposure. The patient should be given an instruction sheet (following) on maintenance and care of the new porcelain laminated veneers.

Patient Instruction Sheet

First 72 Hours

The resin bonding process takes at least 72 hours to cure in its entirety. During this time, you should avoid any hard foods and maintain a relatively soft diet. Extremes in temperature (either hot or cold) should also be avoided. Alcohol and some medicated mouthwashes have the potential to affect the resin bonding material during this early phase and should not be used.

Maintenance

Routine cleanings are a must—at least every four months with a hygienist, who should avoid using an ultrasonic scaler and the air abrasion systems. Use a soft toothbrush with rounded bristles, and floss as you do with natural teeth. If daily cleaning of plaque is a problem, use a mechanical plaque removal device (Interplak, Research Associates, Norcross, Ga.) because plaque-free maintenance of these restorations is essential to their longevity and the health of your teeth and supportive tissues.

Use a less abrasive toothpaste and one that is not highly fluoridated.

Although laminates are strong, avoid excessive biting forces and habit patterns: nail biting, pencil chewing, etc.

Avoid biting into hard pieces of candy, chewing on ice, eating ribs.

Use a soft acrylic mouthguard when involved in any form of contact sport.

Mouthrinses

Acidulated fluoridated mouthrinses can damage the surface finish of your laminates and should be avoided. Chlorhexidine antiplaque mouthrinses may stain your laminates, but the stain can be readily removed by a hygienist.

References

1. Batchelder, K.F., Richter, R.S., and Vaidyanathan, T.K. Can your air compressor affect bond strength? J. Am. Dent. Assoc. 116:203, 205, 1987.

2. Swartz, M.I., Phillips, R.W., and Rhodes, B. Visible light activated resins. Depth of cure. J. Am. Dent. Assoc. 106:209, 1983.

3. Watts, D.C., Amer, O., and Combe, E.C. Characteristics of visible-light-activated composite systems. Br. Dent. J. 156(6):209, 1984.

4. Touati, B. Personal communication, 1985.

Bibliography

Albers, H.F. Tooth Colored Restoratives. 7th ed. Cotati, Calif.: Alto Books, 1985.

Gwinnet, A.J. Bonding factors in techniques which influence clinical success. N.Y. State Dent. J. 48:223, 1982.

Ibsen, R. The New Cosmetic Dentistry Syllabus. Santa Maria, Calif.: Den-Mat Corp., 1987.

Jordan, R.E. Esthetic Composite Bonding. Toronto, Philadelphia: B.C. Decker, 1987.

Nixon, R.L. The Chairside Manual for Porcelain Bonding. Wilmington, Del.: B.A. Videographics, 1987.

Silverstone, L.M., and Dogon, I.L. Proceedings of an International Symposium on the Acid Etch Technique. St. Paul, Minn.: North Central Publishing Co., 1975.

An Atlas of Laminate Placement

Enamel Activation
(Figs. 8-2 to 8-4)

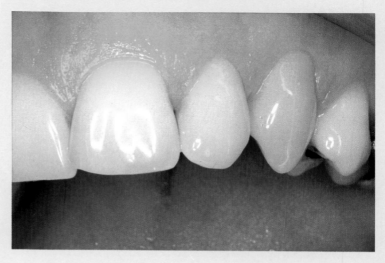

Fig. 8-2 Preoperative view of an esthetically dark canine.

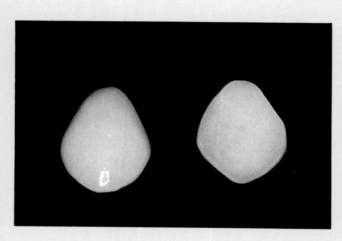

Fig. 8-3 Porcelain laminates as returned from the laboratory. Buccal surface *(left);* etched internal surface *(right).*

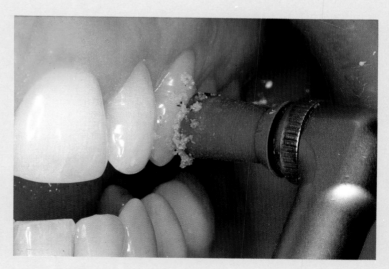

Fig. 8-4 Clean the central incisor of all debris with a slurry of flour of pumice and water.

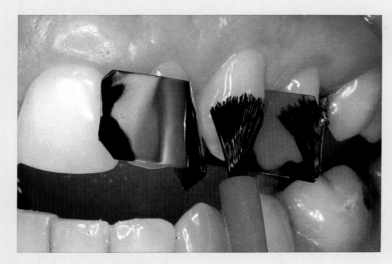

Enamel Etching
(Figs. 8-5 to 8-7)

Fig. 8-5 Isolate the tooth with two dead-soft matrix bands placed mesially and distally and etch the enamel for 15 to 20 seconds.

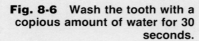 **Fig. 8-6** Wash the tooth with a copious amount of water for 30 seconds.

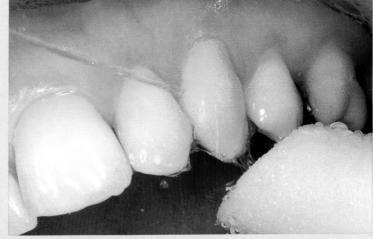

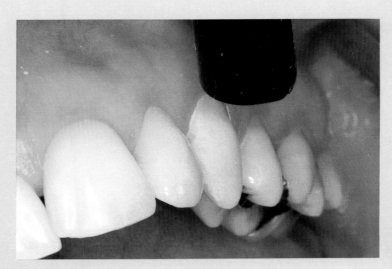

Fig. 8-7 Dry the teeth with an oil-free air syringe and/or utilize a jet of warm air.

Application of Bonding Agent
(Figs. 8-8 to 8-12)

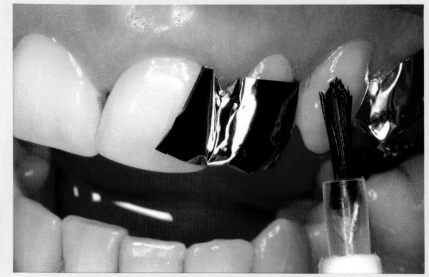

Fig. 8-8 Isolate the tooth once again with dead-soft matrix strips and coat the etched enamel surface with a dentinal bonding agent and/or unfilled resin.

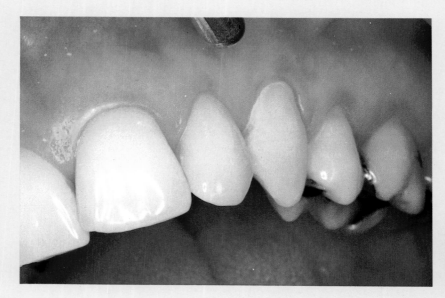

Fig. 8-9 Disperse the bonding agent into a fine, thin layer using a stream of dry air and light cure and seal the surface of the tooth.

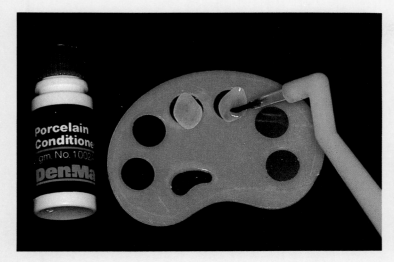

Fig. 8-10 Clean the inner aspect of the veneer with orthophosphoric acid or citric acid. Wash and dry. Drying is further facilitated by coating with a drying agent. Then coat this surface with a layer of silane which is allowed to *evaporate* dry.

Fig. 8-11 Over the dry silane layer, place a layer of unfilled resin. Disperse into a fine layer with a stream of air.

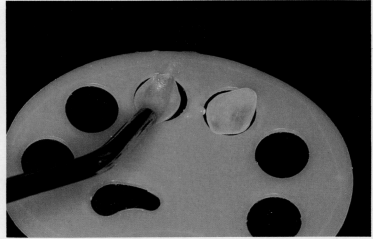

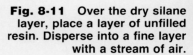

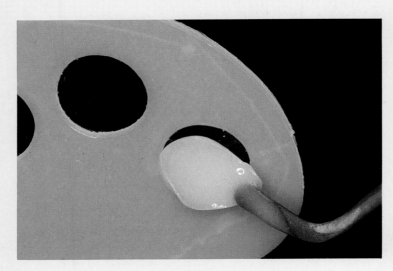

Fig. 8-12 Fill the laminate with the selected composite resin luting agent.

Veneer Placement
(Figs. 8-13 to 8-15)

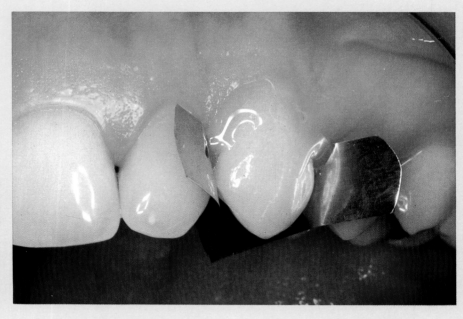

Fig. 8-13 Place the laminate in position on the tooth, rotating it about the incisal edge and towards the gingiva. Ensure that excess luting material exudes from all peripheral aspects of the laminate.

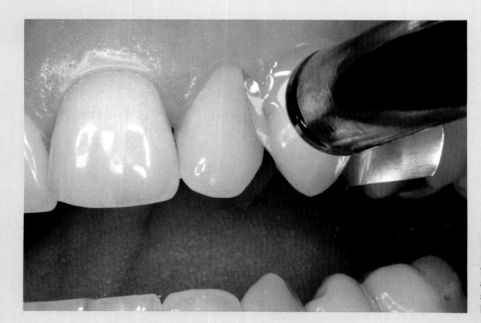

Fig. 8-14 Hold the laminate firmly in place to prevent "suck-back" and light cure for five seconds to tack the laminate in place.

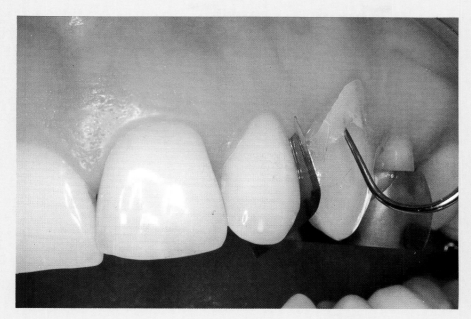

Fig. 8-15 With an explorer or sharp scaler, remove excess, partially surface-cured composite resin that exudes from the laminate margins. Ensure that some composite resin remains in the interface of the laminate and the tooth at the periphery.

Curing
(Fig. 8-16)

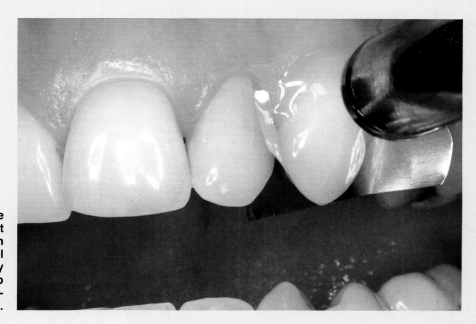

Fig. 8-16 Cure the laminate for at least two minutes on each aspect of the buccal surface and similarly on the lingual. Two lights used simultaneously are preferable.

Finishing
(Figs. 8-17 to 8-24)

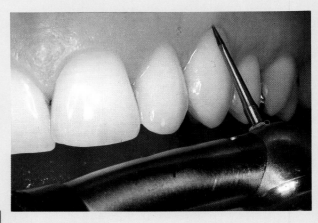

Fig. 8-17 Use carbide finishing bur to remove remaining excess composite resin.

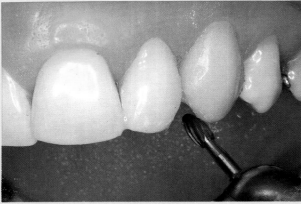

Fig. 8-18 Use the LVS no. 8 diamond to remove composite resin along the incisal lingual margin.

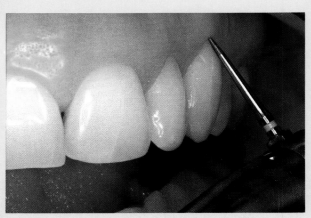

Fig. 8-19 If there is a lateral excessive amount of porcelain beyond the enamel, refine this with a microfine (15 μm) diamond (LVS no. 6) to develop an emergence profile confluent with the original enamel.

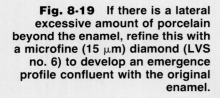

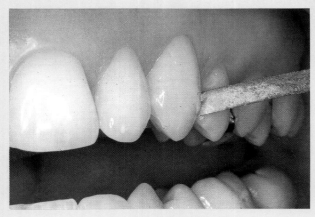

Fig. 8-20 Clear the contacts with an extra-fine metal strip to ensure that they are free.

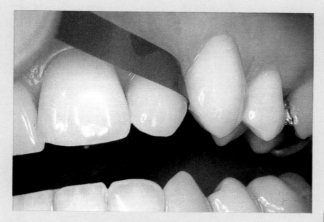

Fig. 8-21 Polish contact areas with composite resin finishing strips.

Fig. 8-22 Polish the tooth/composite resin luting agent/porcelain interface with diamond polishing paste on a nonwebbed rubber cup. Wash and dry.

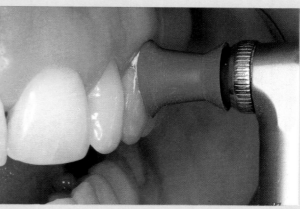

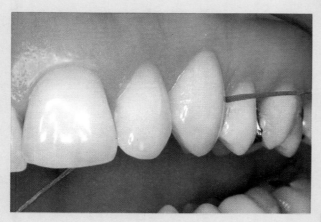

Fig. 8-23 Check interproximal areas for clearance with dental floss.

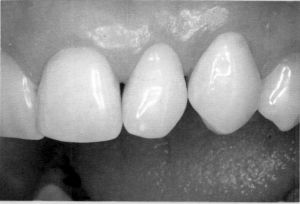

Fig. 8-24 Postoperative view.

Cast Ceramic Laminate Systems

9

There are two distinct systems of cast ceramic laminates:

1. Castable ceramic (Dicor, Dentsply/York Div., York, Pa.)

2. Castable apatite (CeraPearl, Kyocera International, Japan)

The two systems are remarkably similar despite the fact that the procedures and materials are very different. In both, a wax pattern is produced on a conventional working cast and die system. The wax is molded to reproduce the harmonious esthetic tooth form desired (Figs. 9-1 to 9-3). These patterns are finished in their entirety, removed, sprued (Fig. 9-4), and invested (Fig. 9-5) in their respective types of crucibles, depending on the type of system being used.

Each system has its own particular armamentarium, and once the investment is set, the mold is placed in a burn-out furnace and gently heated to volatilize the wax pattern. The crucibles are then correctly heated to the appropriate temperature and placed in their respective casting machines.

For the Dicor system, the cast glass laminate is removed from the investment (Fig. 9-6) and placed in the ceramming oven; this process changes the external surface of the glass and crystalline structure (Figs. 9-7 and 9-8).

For the CeraPearl system, the entire mold is transferred to the crystallization oven and heated at 870°C for one hour. Crystallization takes place, producing a casting of hydroxyapatite crystals. The casting is then separated from the investment and cleaned, using the conventional sand blasting technique with alumina oxide powder.

The cast ceramic laminates can then be smoothed, polished, and tried into the patient's mouth (Fig. 9-9).

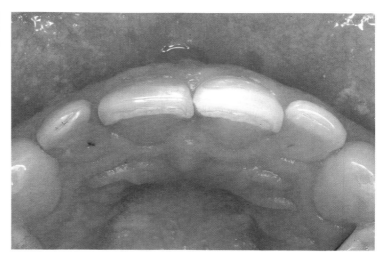

Fig. 9-1 Incisal view showing two lingually located central incisors with striae of discoloration.

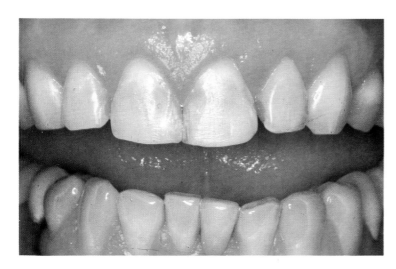

Fig. 9-2 Incisors are prepared for cast glass laminates. Preparation has gingival chamfer and minimal other reduction due to lingual position of the teeth.

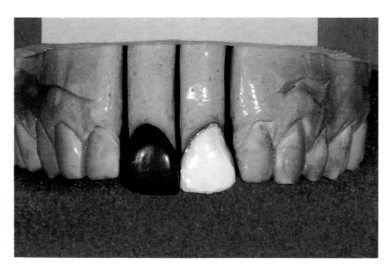

Fig. 9-3 One laminate is waxed to the ideal form on the right central incisor die. The left central incisor die shows a color coordinated die spacer.

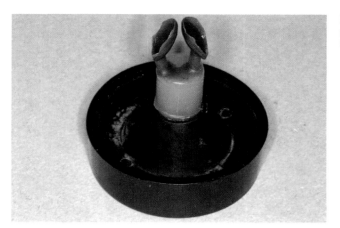

Fig. 9-4 The wax patterns are sprued and ready to be invested.

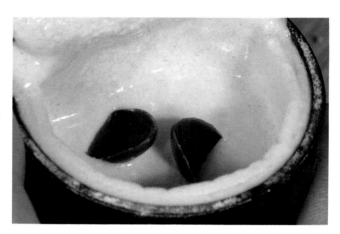

Fig. 9-5 Wax patterns being invested.

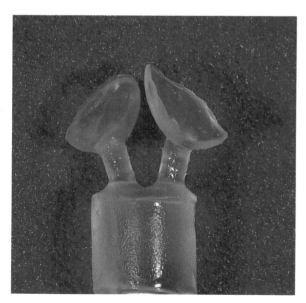

Fig. 9-6 The cast glass laminates after removal from investment.

Fig. 9-7 Cerammed castings following trimming.

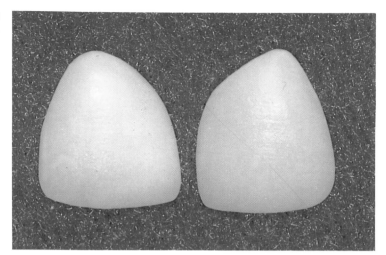

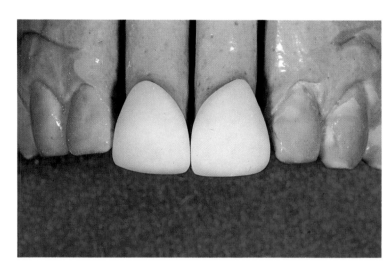

Fig. 9-8 Cerammed castings fitted to dies.

Fig. 9-9 The cerammed castings are tried in for individual fit and contact relations. Any esthetic modifications of tooth form must be completed at this stage.

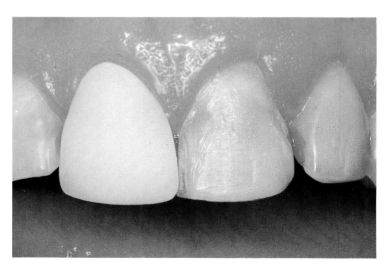

Characterization
(Figs. 9-10 to 9-16)

Shading of the CeraPearl laminates is derived predominately from a resin system that transmits the color from below the hydroxyapatite veneer. Some alteration of the surface can be done with superficial stains.

The external surface of a Dicor laminate is shaded and characterized using the Dicor ceramic shading system and firing it in the conventional manner. Some color modification is also derived from the specific kit of light-activated luting agents, which combines a variety of opaquing and translucent shades. The system also comes with various try-in pastes so that the final shade can be predetermined.

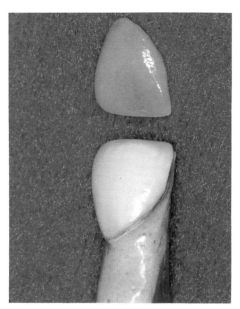

Fig. 9-11 A shaded laminate showing increasing translucency toward the incisal edge. This will be modified by underlying tooth and composite resin luting agent color.

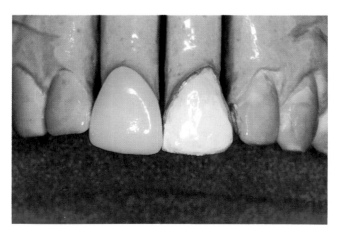

Fig. 9-10 The cerammed castings are shaded.

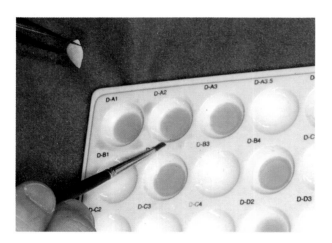

Fig. 9-12 Shaded laminate on the right central incisor die showing the effect of a colored die spacer beneath.

Fig. 9-13 The laminate is filled with appropriate try-in paste.

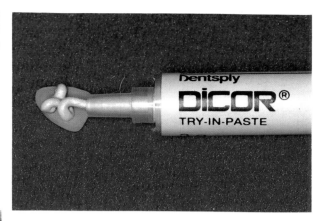

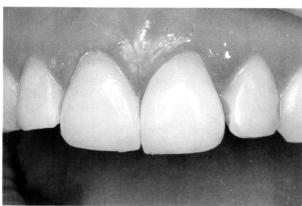

Fig. 9-14 Two laminates are tried in with different colored luting pastes.

Fig. 9-15 The internal surface of laminates are etched.

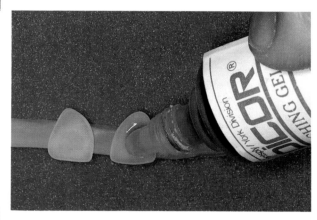

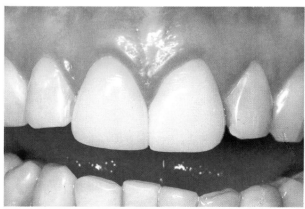

Fig. 9-16 The final laminates are luted in position with a light-cured composite resin.

Enamel Reduction

The enamel reduction required for Dicor and CeraPearl cast ceramic laminates is slightly greater than for conventional baked forms (i.e., 0.6 to 1 mm instead of 0.3 to 0.5 mm).

Etching

These laminate systems are etched internally with different materials. The CeraPearl system uses a 2N hydrochloric acid that selectively erodes the glass matrix. The hydroxyapatite crystals are inert, so the end result is a series of pits and tags on the treated surface, which promotes mechanical adherence.

The Dicor laminate is etched with 10% aluminum difluoride or 10% ammonium.

Advantages

The Dicor and CeraPearl veneers provide particularly intimate fit if the laboratory procedures are correctly performed, and they are the most effective in situations where underlying color of the tooth does not need to be changed too dramatically.

They may also work well in closing small interproximal spaces or small diastemata. If the space between teeth is too large, however, these laminates become difficult to opaque on the unsupported porcelain, which subsequently appears to be gray, due to the dark reflection from the back of the mouth.

The predominant advantage to these two cast ceramic laminate systems appears to be the materials themselves; they are less abrasive than conventional ceramics. CeraPearl is in fact hydroxyapatite, which is a similar substance to enamel composition.

The Dicor material is also less abrasive and closer in properties to the natural tooth enamel. It is, however, covered by a layer of shading porcelain that alters the abrasive nature of the surface. The Dicor laminate also poses a problem should any cosmetic contouring or other adjustment be needed, because the underlying white cerammed glass would be exposed.

Expanded
Clinical
Variations

10

Clinicians have long sought an effective method to replace missing teeth without having to prepare and reduce the adjacent teeth as abutments for fixed partial dentures. The advent of dental adhesive systems initiated the concept of bonding a pontic (such as an acrylic resin denture tooth) in place by utilizing adhesion to the interproximal surfaces of enamel on the tooth adjacent to the space.

Although this was conceived as a useful interim restoration and was obviously a conservative method of maintaining a space and replacing a tooth, it was not always particularly esthetic and obviously not very strong. The very nature of the composite resin material showed cohesive bond strengths that were, for the most part, inadequate to the task, as was the adhesive bond between pontic and luting resin. The strongest point was the resin-enamel bond.

The concept was later expanded so that a porcelain pontic with metal wings on either side con-taining counter-sunk retention holes was bonded to the lingual surface of the adjacent teeth.[1-3] The weak link remained the retainer/resin interface. This improved when Tanaka[4] developed the concept of etching base metal alloys and Livaditas and others[5-8] developed the etched resin retainer for fixed partial dentures. Variations on this type of prosthesis developed in trying to overcome their limitations, but they remained as conservative alternatives to full coverage restorations.[9]

The advent of etching porcelain and bonding it to teeth in the form of veneers[10,11] led ceramists and clinicians to research and develop a system whereby a porcelain pontic in its etched state could be bonded directly to the two adjacent teeth.

Ibsen and Strassler published a paper on the porcelain laminate fixed partial denture whereby porcelain veneers were placed on the buccal surfaces of teeth and carried between them a porcelain pontic; to date, some 1,900 restorations have been placed with about 94% success rate in the anterior part of the arch.[12] Ibsen and Strassler recognized the inordinate advantages of the all-porcelain restoration. They decided to evaluate the natural progression of using porcelain laminate veneers for the single-tooth restoration to using it on the fixed partial denture replacement system. Three basic types of restorations were tried out, as will be discussed.

Conventional Lingual-Etched Porcelain Retainers

In the case of conventional lingual-etched porcelain retainers, a Rochette[1] style restoration replacing the maxillary right lateral incisor (Figs.

10-1a and b) was removed. Lingual clearance had been developed for the use of the metal retainers and it was decided to use a similar pattern with etched porcelain for the wings. The existing preparations were rounded out and smoothed (Fig. 10-1c) and a definitive cingulum rest on both teeth was developed. The interproximal modification was limited to developing as much enamel contact as possible without altering the esthetics but providing for a single path of insertion. The fixed partial denture was fabricated according to techniques described in chapter 7 (Fig. 10-1d). The try-in and bonding procedure is the same as that for conventional placement of laminates, as is the finishing. The final restoration (Figs. 10-1e and f) is adjusted so that no contact is made on the pontic during excursive movement of the mandible.

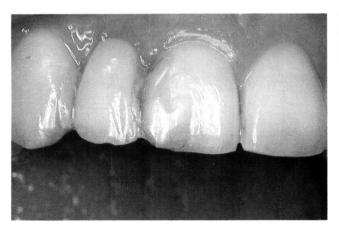

Fig. 10-1a This case shows an old, discolored, Rochette style fixed partial denture to be replaced.

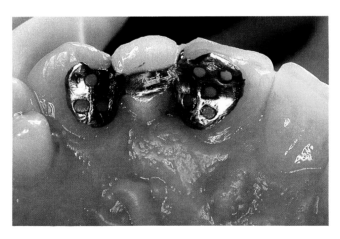

Fig. 10-1b Lingual view.

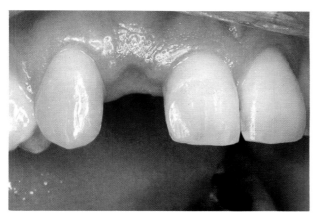

Fig. 10-1c Preparation for etched porcelain restoration.

Fig. 10-1d The etched porcelain restoration showing lingual retention wings and a pontic.

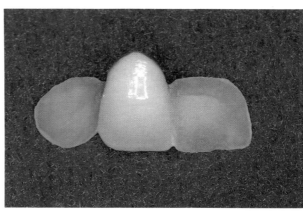

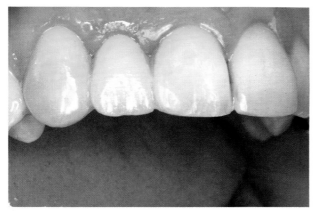

Fig. 10-1e The etched porcelain restoration luted in position.

Fig. 10-1f Linguoincisal view of restoration bonded in place.

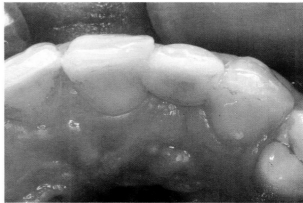

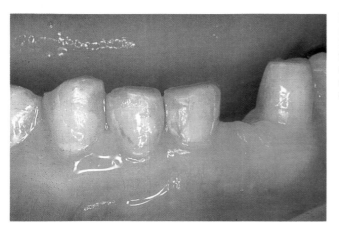

Fig. 10-2a Postorthodontic view of a young woman showing missing left lateral incisor, a right canine in the position of a right lateral incisor, and the first premolar in the position of the canine. The teeth are worn and discolored.

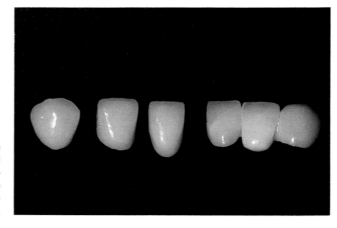

Fig. 10-2b The porcelain laminate restoration: a pontic with labioincisal veneers and three individual laminates to convert the right canine into a lateral incisor and the first premolar into a canine.

Buccal-Etched Porcelain Retainers

In this case the dramatic advantage of porcelain laminate veneers over any other form of etched retainer is immediately evident. The young woman seen in Fig. 10-2a had missing mandibular lateral incisors. Following orthodontics, the teeth were in relative position but somewhat broken down. A gingivectomy and a ridge augmentation in the mandibular anterior sextant were performed to increase tooth length and provide for soft tissue health and esthetics. The laminates that were placed on the buccal surface of the teeth improved the esthetics of these teeth as well as increased their length in order to develop occlusal function with the maxillary anterior teeth. The fixed partial denture extended from the left mandibular canine to the left central incisor—carrying a pontic to replace the lateral incisor (Fig. 10-2b).

The preparation for this case involved reducing the incisal edge, rounding the buccoincisal line angle, and developing a mini-chamfer on the linguoincisal line angle. The labial surface was reduced 0.3 mm with the development of a modified chamfer confluent with the gingival margin. In addition, the right central incisor was prepared for a single laminate and the right canine was reduced so that a laminate could be fabricated to simulate a lateral incisor. The right first premolar was prepared to receive a laminate to simulate a right canine. The bonding and placement procedures, as described previously, were used to provide a conservative, functional, and most esthetic fixed partial denture (Figs. 10-2c and d).

Fig. 10-2c The completed prosthesis, labial view.

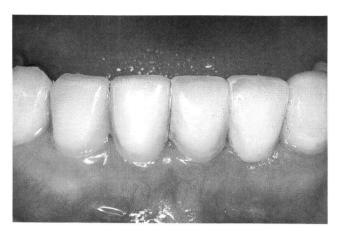

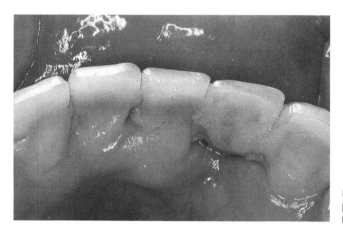

Fig. 10-2d The lingual view of the prosthesis shows pontic and laminates with incisal coverage.

Combination Buccal and Lingual Retainers

A young man had congenitally missing lateral incisors, and an ineffectual overjet and lingual clearance (Fig. 10-3a). The placement of lingual-supporting porcelain would redevelop premolar guidance. In addition, the teeth were canted somewhat lingually and for esthetic purposes needed to be brought out labially. There was a diastema between the two central incisors.

Fabrication of the fixed partial denture involved a complete wraparound of the premolar on both the buccal and lingual surfaces with a lingual retainer on the central incisor (Fig. 10-3b). In addition, to round out the arch and close the diastema, two separate central incisor laminates

were fabricated (Fig. 10-3c). The prosthesis was placed in two separate stages—the partial denture was placed first and then the two central incisor laminates were placed, following curing and finishing.

This case shows the enormous versatility of the procedures. Without any reduction of the tooth surface whatsoever, and by utilizing supragingival margins, this patient was provided with an esthetic tooth replacement and his canine guidance returned to normal (Figs. 10-3d to g).

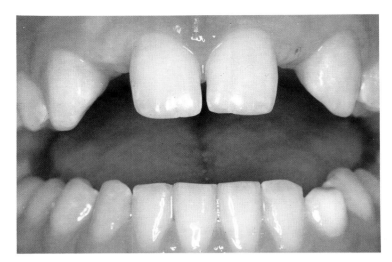

Fig. 10-3a This patient had congenitally missing lateral incisors, spacing, and inadequate anterior guidance.

Fig. 10-3b The etched porcelain restoration shows complete wraparound of the canine and a lingual wing on the central incisor.

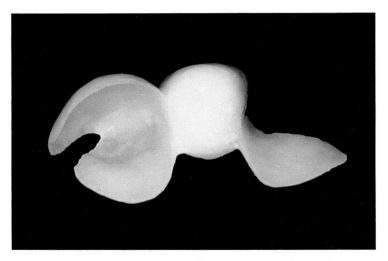

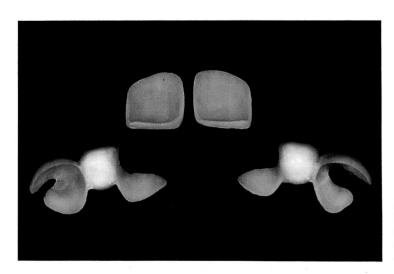

Fig. 10-3c Two etched porcelain restorations and two individual central incisor laminates to close the disastema and round out the arch form.

Fig. 10-3d Labial view of the bonded prosthesis.

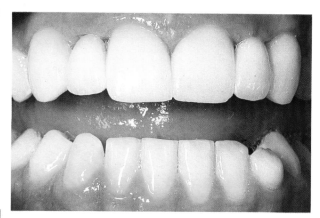

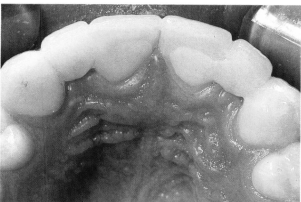

Fig. 10-3e The lingual view of the prosthesis shows canine guidance developed with the etched porcelain wing. The wing on the central incisor is located below the contact area of the mandibular incisors.

Fig. 10-3f Smile line prior to lateral incisor replacement.

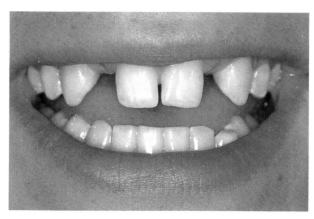

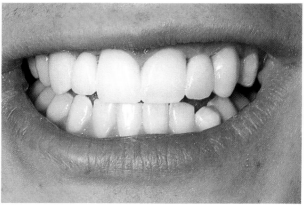

Fig. 10-3g Smile line restored with no reduction of tooth structure and etched porcelain veneer restoration.

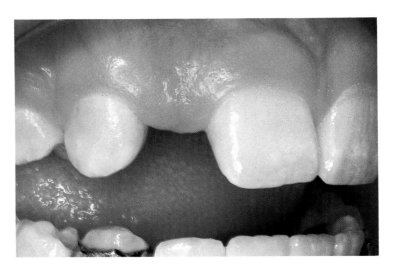

Fig. 10-4a Preoperative view showing congenitally missing lateral incisor.

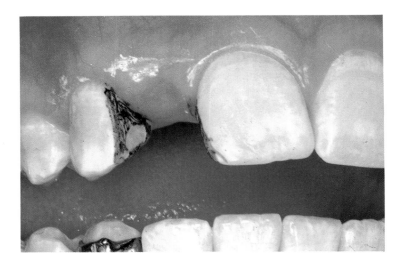

Fig. 10-4b Preparation stage. A Class III type of preparation within the confines of the green shaded area.

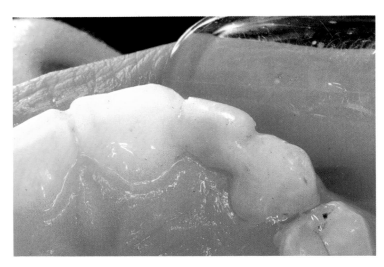

Fig. 10-4c Lingual view of interproximal retainer type of etched porcelain fixed partial denture.

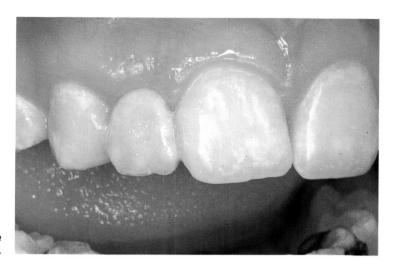

Fig. 10-4d Buccal view of the restoration bonded into position.

Interproximal Retainers

If the abutment teeth are esthetically pleasing and not compromised by previous restorations, then the preparation may be limited solely to the adjacent interproximal regions. This is basically a rounded, shallow, interproximal, Class III type of preparation. It should extend in an apicocoronal dimension from 0.5 mm above the soft tissue to 0.5 mm short of the rounded proximal corner of the incisal edge.

In a buccolingual dimension, it begins 0.5 mm beyond the buccoproximal line angle—extending around onto the lingual surface for 2 to 3 mm. Interproximal areas are modified to facilitate a single path of insertion and to develop increased surface area for increased retention. The lingual Class III cavities are about 0.7 mm deep and well rounded apart from the vertical stop on the apical aspect of the preparation. The preparations must remain entirely in enamel for maximum retention and allow for an increased thickness of porcelain in the interproximal bonding areas where stress concentrations will be highest.

It should be noted that these restorations are still experimental in nature and very much depend on the fracture resistance of the porcelain. New reinforced ceramic systems will move them out of the experimental realm into everyday practice, but in the interim, they should be used judiciously on very select cases for single-tooth replacement (Figs. 10-4a to d).

Etched Porcelain "Pieces"

The strength and esthetics of the porcelain laminate can be utilized to effectively close small spaces and diastemata. The enamel of teeth in these situations is just roughened up somewhat, so that the laboratory technician has a nominal thickness on which to build the porcelain. The porcelain is fabricated in such a way that it has maximum opacity in the area where the space existed; translucency is built in step-wise toward the proximal edge (Fig. 10-5a). The porcelain is matched identically to the tooth shade, and the composite resin that is used should be of a relatively translucent nature so that the underlying color of the tooth will blend through the resin and the more translucent porcelain at the edge of the restoration, making the junction between tooth, resin, and porcelain indistinguishable (Figs. 10-5b and c).

Accurate location of the porcelain "piece" during placement is difficult because there is no definitive seat. By using a light-cured resin the chip can be moved into position and then lightly tacked into place so that it can be checked prior to final curing. The rest of the procedure is, for the most part, identical to full laminate placement. The great advantage is maintenance of the integrity of the tooth structure as well as the lifelike esthetics, strength, and durability of porcelain.

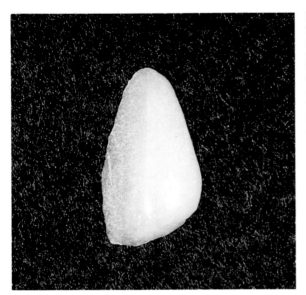

Fig. 10-5a An etched porcelain "chip" to fill in a space between a lateral incisor and a canine. Note the opacity of the porcelain on the uppermost aspect, which will fill in the space between the teeth; this is blended out with translucent porcelain toward the opposite edge. This allows for the color of the tooth to blend through to make for an indistinguishable junction.

Fig. 10-5b Space between lateral incisor and canine.

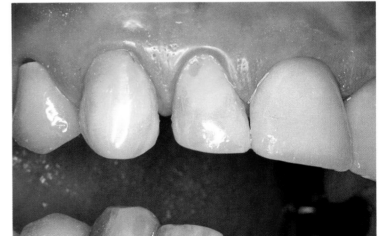

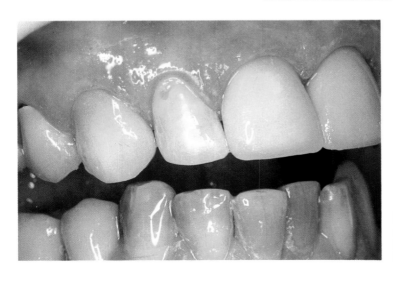

Fig. 10-5c Space filled by porcelain chip, restoring lifelike esthetics and function with durability of porcelain.

References

1. Rochette, A.L. Attachment of a splint to enamel of lower anterior teeth. J. Prosthet. Dent. 30:418–423, 1973.

2. Howe, D.F., and Denehy, G.E. Anterior fixed partial denture utilizing the acid-etch technique and a cast metal framework. J. Prosthet. Dent. 37:28–31, 1977.

3. Kuhlke, K.L., and Drennon, D.G. An alternative to the anterior single-tooth removable partial denture. J. Int. Assoc. Dental Child. 8:11–14, 1977.

4. Tanaka, T., et al. Pitting corrosion for retaining acrylic resin facings. J. Prosthet. Dent. 42:282–291, 1979.

5. Livaditis, G.J. Cast metal resin-bonded retainers for posterior teeth. J. Am. Dent. Assoc. 101:926–929, 1980.

6. Thompson, V.P., and Livaditis, G.J. Etched casting acid etch composite bonded posterior bridges. Pediatric Dent. 4(1):38–43, 1982.

7. Denehy, G.E. Use of acid etch composites in anterior bridge construction. Pediatric Dent. 4(1):44–47, 1982.

8. Eshleman, J.R., et al. Retentive strength of acid etched fixed prostheses. J. Dent. Res. 60(Spec. Issue A):349, 1981.

9. Rochette, A.L. Les bondlags moyen d'ancrage en prosthèse fixée—14 ans de recal. St. Paul, Minn.: 3M Company, 1975.

10. Horn, H.R. Porcelain laminate veneers bonded to etched enamel. Dent. Clin. North Am. 27:671, 1983.

11. Calamia, J.R. Etched porcelain facial veneers: a new treatment modality. N.Y. J. Dent. 53:255–259, 1983.

12. Ibsen, R.L., and Strassler, H.E. An innovative method for fixed anterior tooth replacement utilizing porcelain veneers. Quintessence Int. 17:455, 1986.

Indirect Composite Resin Veneers: An Alternative

11

Harald O. Heymann

In recent years, laboratory processed composite resins have been developed not only for use as restorative materials in fixed prosthodontics, but also as indirect veneering materials. Using light, heat, vacuum, or a combination thereof, microfilled resin materials can be processed to achieve physical and mechanical properties superior to those of traditional chairside composite resins. Even though the inorganic filler content is relatively low, ranging from 30% to 50% by weight,[1] studies indicate that the wear resistance of these materials is surprisingly good.[2-4] Through laboratory processing, indirect resin veneers are more completely cured and do not experience the same in situ polymerization problems typically encountered during conventional direct composite resin veneering.

Fabrication of *direct* composite resin veneers are quite time consuming and present a significant shortcoming: they are technique-sensitive and depend on the operator's artistic ability and attention to detail. *Indirect* composite resin veneers are typically fabricated by a trained technician, and so less effort is required by the dentist in achieving the final contours of the restoration. They therefore usually require less overall clinical chair time.[5]

Unlike prefabricated acrylic resin laminates composed of a polymethyl methacrylate resin, indirect composite resin veneers are closely related in composition to chairside composite resins. Therefore, indirect veneers of this type are inherently capable of achieving chemical bonding to the composite resin bonding medium, with no pretreatment of the veneer required. Indirectly fabricated composite resin veneers offer advantages of superior shading capabilities and control of facial contours. Also, because they are composed of microfilled resins, they can be polished to a lustrous finish.

Although indirect composite resin veneers offer many advantages over direct resin veneers, their limited bond strength restricts their use to cases not involving heavy functional contacts.

Clinical Technique

These veneers are indirectly fabricated by a laboratory and so require two patient appointments: one for preparation of the teeth and the securing of an elastomeric impression, and the second for bonding and finishing the veneers.

Both extraenamel and intraenamel veneering techniques are possible. Although extraenamel approaches are less invasive, there is a tendency toward increased tooth thickness and bulbous contours. Intraenamel preparations provide a definite finish line to compensate for the thickness of the veneering material,[6-10] providing better tooth contours and hence good gingival health.

In the case chosen to illustrate this technique, defective direct composite resin veneers were originally present (Fig. 11-1). Visio-Gem (ESPE-Premier, Valley Stream, N.Y.), was used as the indirect veneering material.

Shade selection is determined prior to isolation of the teeth in order to eliminate shading variations that can occur because of drying and dehydration of the teeth. Both body and incisal shades of composite resin are available, as are characterizing resins for optional esthetic modifications.

Following shade selection, the teeth are isolated with the use of bilaterally placed absorbent cotton rolls and gingival retraction cord. A small-diameter retraction cord, atraumatically placed in the labial gingival sulcus, provides improved access and visibility during preparation of the teeth. All existing defective Class III restorations or small carious lesions should be replaced or restored prior to initiating the veneer preparations.

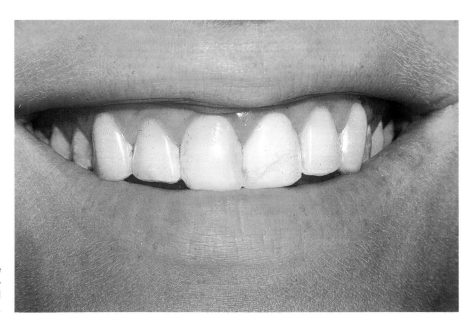

Fig. 11-1 Defective composite resin veneers to be replaced by indirect veneers.

The teeth to be veneered are prepared with a round or bevel-ended diamond stone to a depth approximately equivalent to half the enamel thickness. The depth of reduction typically ranges from 0.5 to 0.6 mm midfacially, to 0.2 to 0.3 mm along the gingival aspect of the preparation. Greater reduction may be required if significant intrinsic staining exists, as in cases involving severe tetracycline staining. Ideally, however, the entire preparation should be restricted to enamel to allow acid-etching for micromechanical retention.

Reduction may be gauged by using either depth cuts or a hemi-preparation technique. A no. 1/4 round bur, typically 0.4 mm in diameter, is well suited for depth gauging. The hemi-preparation technique allows inspection of the remaining unprepared tooth structure in cross section following preparation of only one half of the facial surface.

A moderate chamfer should be created along the margins of the preparation. The interproximal margins should be extended beyond the interproximal line angles of the tooth yet be positioned labial to the contact areas. The gingival margin is prepared at a level equal to that of the free gingival crest. *Subgingival extension of the prepared margins should be avoided.* Incisally, the preparation should be restricted to the facial aspect of the incisal edge and should never be terminated in an area subjected to occlusal function. In these situations, or if a tooth requires lengthening, indirect composites resin veneers are not recommended. The completed preparations are illustrated in Fig. 11-2.

An elastomeric impression of the prepared teeth is generated following removal of the retraction cord. Because the preparation is restricted to enamel, it is not noticeably objec-

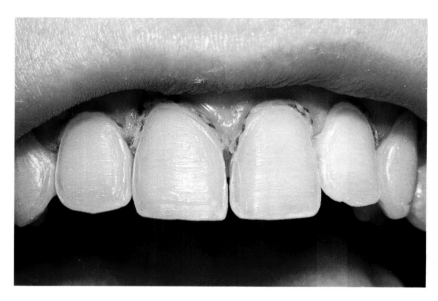

Fig. 11-2 Completed tooth preparation shows tissue displacement cord in place.

tionable to the patient, and no temporization is required.

A working cast with individually removable dies of the prepared teeth is fabricated and forwarded to the laboratory. Removable dies are recommended to allow the technician complete access to interproximal areas. Once the completed composite resin veneers are returned, they should be inspected for fracture lines, chips, or other significant defects that would preclude successful placement.

At the second appointment, the basic placement process for composite resin veneers is similar to that described in chapter 8 for porcelain veneers, with some minor differences. The prepared teeth are first thoroughly cleaned with a flour of pumice or an oil- and fluoride-free cleansing paste.

The teeth are once again isolated with bilateral cotton rolls. Gingival retraction cord is placed in the labial gingival sulcus to retract the tissue and reduce seepage of the gingival fluids.

To evaluate veneer fit, a try-in of each veneer is recommended. Minor adjustments to the veneer can still be made with suitable composite resin finishing burs or diamonds to enhance adaptation.

Some manufacturers of indirect resin veneers offer a light-cured bonding medium specifically produced for use with their veneers. Typically, these bonding media are simply more fluid versions of a preexisting composite resin. If no separate bonding resin is available, a bonding medium can be created by blending a small amount of unfilled resin with an appropriate shade of composite resin. In the case illustrated, Visio-Fil (ESPE-Premier, Valley Stream, N.Y.), a light-cured conventional composite resin, was blended with Visio-Bond (ESPE-Premier), an unfilled fluid resin, to produce the bonding medium. The two components consisted of 75% by weight Visio-Fil and 25% by weight Visio-Bond (approximately 6 mm of Visio-Fil as dispensed from the manufacturer's syringe per drop of Visio-Bond). The mixture is vigorously blended in a dappen dish until a honey-like consistency suitable for bonding is attained.

The shade of composite resin used in the mixture is that which most closely resembles the shade of the veneer. However, upon trial positioning the veneers, it may be discovered that slight shade modifications are required. Minor es-

thetic changes can be achieved simply by incorporating a small amount of color modifier into the mixture or by applying the modifier directly to the inner aspect of the veneer prior to placement.

In order to optimize moisture control, the teeth are isolated and etched and the veneers are placed one by one.

If the inner aspect of the veneer is totally smooth, a coarse diamond stone should be used to *lightly* roughen the underside of the veneer, thus improving the potential for additional micromechanical bonding. This step is particularly important if there has been no intraenamel preparation, when the inner aspect of the veneer will be smooth. Care must also be taken not to inadvertently contaminate the underside of the veneer prior to bonding. If the inner aspect of the veneer is touched, it should be cleaned with acetone or ethyl alcohol prior to bonding so as to remove any oils or surface contaminants.

A thin film of the unfilled resin bonding agent is placed on the etched enamel but not yet cured. The veneer is then loaded with a homogeneous layer of the Visio-Fil/Visio-Bond blend, approximately 0.5 mm thick, and is seated on the tooth. The veneer should be positioned first at the gingival margin, allowing the excess cement to extrude incisally as the veneer is fully seated. Caution must be exercised not to entrap air between the tooth and veneer. The intraenamel preparation acts as a guide for indexing and positioning the veneer. However, prior to polymerization, the veneer should be held firmly in place while an explorer is used to check for marginal adaptation. Excess bonding medium can be removed with an explorer or composite resin instrument at this time.

The underlying bonding medium is polymerized for at least 40 seconds with a visible light-curing unit from both facial and lingual directions. If a layer of opaque resin has been incorporated into the resin veneer, this curing time should be at least doubled.

Following complete polymerization, excess bonding material is removed using conventional composite resin finishing burs and instruments. Removal of the gingival retraction cord at this time facilitates access and visibility for finishing procedures. A combination of 12- and 30-fluted flame-shaped composite resin finishing burs or micron finishing diamonds work well for finishing and smoothing facial areas. Portions of the ve-

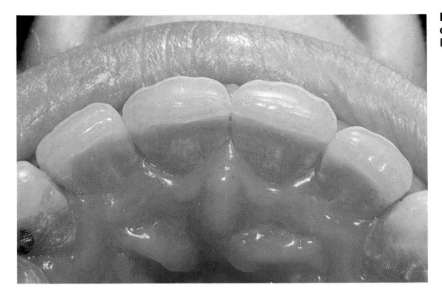

Fig. 11-3 Incisal view of the completed resin laminates.

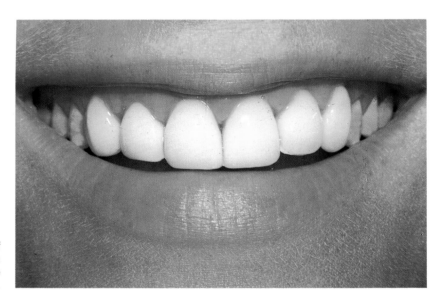

Fig. 11-4 Facial view of the laminates luted in position. Premolars were subsequently veneered.

neer roughened by finishing procedures can be further smoothed and polished to a lustrous surface using abrasive disks and points. Command Ultrafine Luster Paste (Kerr/Sybron, Romulus, Mich.) is recommended for imparting a final enamel-like surface luster.

The completed veneers are shown in Figs. 11-3 and 11-4. Note that the incisal edges are maintained in enamel to protect the veneer from shearing forces experienced during protrusive excursions.

Following bonding of all veneers, the occlusion must be evaluated to ensure that no functional interferences have been introduced. Protrusive and lateral functional contacts should be restricted to enamel if at all possible.

Clinical Observations

Based on two years of clinical observations,[11] it appears that indirectly fabricated resin veneers can offer a viable and esthetic alternative to directly applied composite resin veneers. However, some minor clinical deficiencies have become apparent.

First, the surface glaze of unfilled resin that is typically polymerized on the facial surface of the veneer wears away within the first year. A highly lustrous surface, however, can be reestablished through conventional chairside finishing and polishing techniques as described earlier. For this reason, surface glazing by the laboratory is not recommended. A more permanent and durable surface luster is attained if the operator simply finishes and polishes the veneer immediately following bonding.

Second, indirectly fabricated resin veneers are somewhat prone to chipping and fracture when subjected to excessive functional or biting forces. According to a study conducted by Jordan and others involving over 100 Visio-Gem and Dentacolor (Kulzer, Inc., Irvine, Calif.) veneers, 16% experienced chipping or cohesive fracture after one year of recalls.[12] Therefore, case selection appears critical to the long-term clinical success of these veneers. As alluded to earlier, indirect resin veneers should not be subjected to heavy occlusal stresses.

Bond Strength

The two bonding interfaces that are involved with the resin bonding medium are the inner surface of the processed composite resin veneer and the acid-etched enamel. The bond strength of composite resin to etched enamel has been well documented. Tensile bond strengths ranging from 2,000 psi (140 kg/cm^2) to 2,750 psi (192 kg/cm^2) have been reported.[13-15] By comparison, the highest tensile bond strengths for the bonding medium (Visio-Fil/Visio-Bond blend) to processed resin veneers of Visio-Gem and Dentacolor have been reported to be 1,480 psi (103 kg/cm^2) and 1,391 psi (97 kg/cm^2) respectively.[16] Owing to this fact, the weaker of the two interfaces appears to be the resin veneer/bonding agent interface. This interface has also been reported to be the most frequent site of failure in acrylic laminate veneers.[17,18] Therefore, as stated earlier, indirect composite resin veneers should be restricted for use in areas not subjected to significant functional forces that may chip or fracture the veneers.

Etched porcelain veneers treated with a silane coupling agent seem to offer bond strengths more closely approaching that of etched enamel, exhibiting an average tensile bond strength of 2,083 psi (146 kg/cm^2).[18,19] Even greater shear bond strengths approaching 3,500 psi have been reported.[20] As evidenced by these research reports, *etched porcelain veneers appear to provide significantly greater retentive strength* to etched enamel than that which is attainable with indirect composite resin veneers.

According to a recent study by Heymann and others, the bonding mechanism for indirect composite resin veneers most likely involves a combination of chemical adhesion and micromechanical retention.[21] Because of the processing procedures involved in fabricating an indirect composite resin veneer, the degree of polymerization is significantly greater than that achieved by conventional chairside in situ polymerization techniques. Therefore, the potential for establishing strong chemical bonds between the processed veneer and the resin bonding medium is significantly diminished. Much of the interfacial bonding that occurs is most likely micromechanical in nature. Thus, a bonding medium that can readily flow and wet the substrate is all important. However, assuming some chemical bonding does occur, it is vital that the laboratory turnaround time for veneer fabrication be held to a minimum. Related studies show that the potential for chemical bonding decreases with the age of the composite resin.[22] *Therefore, veneer bonding should occur as soon after fabrication of the veneers as possible.*

Porcelain Versus Resin Veneers

Although significant overlap occurs regarding the clinical indications for porcelain and resin veneers, case selection largely determines which indirect veneering system is most appropriate. The advantages and disadvantages of each sys-

Table 11-1 Summary of various clinical characteristics and relative advantages of porcelain versus resin veneers

Characteristic	Porcelain	Resin
Retention/strength	√	
Surface texture	√	
Lab fee		√
Longevity	√	
Repairability		√
Ease of replacement		√

tem must be weighed and considered when deciding on the course of treatment. A summary of the various clinical characteristics along with the apparent relative strengths of each indirect veneering system is presented in Table 11-1.

Based on studies previously cited, it is evident that superior veneer strength and retention are possible with etched porcelain veneers. For this important reason, etched porcelain veneers appear to be a more prudent restorative alternative in cases requiring significant lengthening of teeth or involving functional occlusal contacts. However, the bond strength of indirect resin veneers seems to be adequate for some routine circumstances not involving functional forces.

The surface texture of glazed porcelain is also superior to that of polished resin because of its durability and high luster. However, in areas where the veneer surface is disturbed by contouring and finishing, it is significantly more difficult to reestablish a highly polished surface to porcelain veneers than to resin.

Resin veneers typically incur one third to one half the laboratory charges of porcelain veneers. However, porcelain veneers, which are seemingly more durable than resin veneers, may require less frequent replacement, resulting in long-term cost savings.

Due to their composition, indirect resin veneers are easily matched and repaired with chairside, light-cured microfilled resins. They are also more easily replaced than are porcelain veneers. If the original master cast is retained, a new resin veneer can be produced for immediate bonding following removal of the defective veneer. Replacement of porcelain veneers usually requires two appointments because of the difficulty in removing the defective veneer without altering the original intraenamel preparation. It should be noted, however, that the need for repair or replacement is apparently less with porcelain veneers because of their superior bond strength and retention to etched enamel.

Intraenamel veneers of processed composite resin are currently being used for the esthetic restoration of generalized facial stains or defects. Because these veneers are fabricated indirectly, they possess physical properties superior to chairside microfilled resins and are less technique-sensitive to operator ability. Although the bond strength of indirect resin veneers is not as great as that of etched porcelain veneers, the minimal cost, simplicity of fabrication, and esthetic qualities of indirect resin veneers make them a viable alternative to other veneering systems in certain selected cases.

References

1. Farah, J.W., and Powers, J.M. (eds.) Report on resin veneers. Dent. Advisor 2(4):7, 1985.

2. Michl, R.J. Isosit—a new dental material. Quintessence Int. 9(3):29–33, 1978.

3. Phillips, R.W. Symposium report. p. 3 *In* Official Precis of the First International Symposium on the Clinical Applications of Light-Cured Composites. Valley Stream, N.Y.: ESPE-Premier Sales Corp., 1985.

4. Oberlander, E. A new light-curing crown and bridge veneering material. Clinical report. Quintessence Int. 15:471–476, 1984.

5. Heymann, H.O. Symposium report. p. 4 *In* Official Precis of the First International Symposium on the Clinical Applications of Laboratory Light-Cured Composites. Valley Stream, N.Y.: ESPE-Premier Sales Corp., 1985.

6. Black, J.B. Esthetic restoration of tetracycline-stained teeth. J. Am. Dent. Assoc. 104:846–852, 1982.

7. Sockwell, C.L., Heymann, H.O., and Brunson, W.D. Additional conservative and esthetic treatments. pp. 312–372 *In* C.M. Sturdevant (ed.) The Art and Science of Operative Dentistry. St. Louis: The C. V. Mosby Co., 1985.

8. Jordan, R.E., Suzuki, M., and Gwinnett, A.J. Conservative applications of acid etch-resin techniques. Dent. Clin. North Am. 25:307–336, 1981.

9. Black, J.B. Morphological effect of enamel reduction on bonded veneers. N.Y. State Dent. J. 51:644–646, 1985.

10. Gross, J.S., and Malcmacher, L.J. An improved color coordination system for indirect veneers. Quintessence Int. 16:707–711, 1985.

11. Heymann, H.O. Indirect composite resin veneers: clinical technique and two-year observations. Quintessence Int. 17:111–118, 1987.

12. Boksman, L. Customized laminate veneers, porcelain and composite. *In* J.W. Clark (ed.) Clinical Dentistry. Vol. 4. Philadelphia: J.B. Lippincott Co., 1986.

13. Bowen, R.L. A method for bonding to dentin and enamel. J. Am. Dent. Assoc. 107:734–736, 1983.

14. Laswell, H.R., Welk, D.A., and Regenos, J.W. Attachment of resin restorations to acid pretreated enamel. J. Am. Dent. Assoc. 82:558–563, 1971.

15. Council on Dental Materials, Instruments, and Equipment. Resin dentin bonding systems. J. Am. Dent. Assoc. 108:240–241, 1984.

16. Nicholls, J.I. Esthetic veneer cementation. J. Prosthet. Dent. 56:9–12, 1986.

17. Boyer, D.B., and Chalkley, Y. Bonding between acrylic laminates and composite resin. J. Dent. Res. 61:489–492, 1982.

18. Calamia, J.R. Etched porcelain veneers: the current state of the art. Quintessence Int. 16:5–12, 1985.

19. Calamia, J.R., and Simonsen, R.J. Effect of coupling agents on bond strength of etched porcelain. J. Dent. Res. 63:179(Abstr. no. 79), 1984.

20. Hsu, C.S., Stangel, I., and Nathanson, D. Shear bond strength of resin to etched porcelain. J. Dent. Res. 64:296(Abstr. no. 1095), 1985.

21. Heymann, H.O., et al. Bonding agent strengths with processed composite resin veneers. Dent. Mat. 3(3):121–124, 1987.

22. Boyer, D.B., Chan, K.C., and Reinhardt, J.W. Build-up and repair of light-cured composites: bond strength. J. Dent. Res. 63:1241–1244, 1984.

Index

impression
    preparation 63
    preparation 62

P

Patient instruction
  sheet 98
Platinum foil
  technique, 67–76
  die preparation 67,
    68, 69
  foil choice 67
  foil matrix 67, 70, 71,
    72, 73
  foil removal 76
  model preparation 67
Porcelain,
  bond strength 26, 28,
    30, 31, 32
  buildup, 67, 73, 74,
    75, 76
    conventional 83
    for tooth
      discoloration
      83–88
    for tooth root 84, 85
    incisal effects 86,
      87, 88
    P.A. Opacity
      System 83, 84,
      88, 89
    "piano keys" 86, 89
  light transmission 32,
    33
  longevity of
    restorations 34
  strengthening 24–34
  technology 24–35
  thickness effect on
    bond strength 32,
    33
Porcelain, etched,
  bond strength 26, 28,
    30, 31, 32
  characteristics 25
  etching time effect 26
  resin interface 26, 29
  solution effects 26, 27
  surface 25, 30

Porcelain, unetched,
  bond strength 26, 28
  resin interface 26, 29
  surface 25, 30

R

Refractory investment
  technique 61–66
Restorations,
  longevity of
    porcelain 34
  unesthetic, veneers
    for 20

S

Shear bond strength
  test 26, 28, 30, 31
Sulcular extension 41,
  49

T

Temporization 54
Tetracycline stains 41
Tooth,
  agenesis, veneers
    for 20, 22
  aging, veneers for 20,
    21
  discoloration,
    tetracycline 41
    veneers for 16, 17,
      83–88
  fractures (Class IV),
    veneers for 88, 89
  malpositioned, veneers
    for 17, 19, 20, 21
  wear, veneers for 20,
    21
Tooth preparation,
  enamel reduction
    36–51
  for porcelain laminate
    veneers 36, 54, 56
  tissue
    displacement 53

V

Veneer,
  bonding 11
  history of 11–13
Veneer, acrylic 56–58
Veneer, cast ceramic
  laminate, 108–114
  advantages 114
  castable apatite 108
  castable ceramic 108
  ceramming 108, 110,
    111
  characterizing 112,
    113
  wax pattern 108, 109,
    110
Veneer, composite resin,
  direct 54
  direct-vacuform
    matrix 55, 56, 57
  indirect, 57, 127–133
    bond strength 131
    clinical
      observations 131
    clinical
      technique
      127–130
    intraenamel 132
    porcelain veneer
      compared 131, 132
Veneer, porcelain
  laminate,
  advantages 15, 22
  characterizing 82–89,
    93
  color, 91
  color check 91
  contouring 76, 98
  contraindications 23
  disadvantages 15, 22
  esthetics 98
  etched "pieces" 123,
    124
  etching 77, 78
  fabrication
    techniques 60,
      61–66, 67–76
  features 14–23
  finishing 76, 97, 106,
    107